Exam Success Review

MCQ's for MBBS 1st Prof & PG Entrance

ANATOMY

Abdomen & Lower Limb

Volume - 3

Dr. Brijendra Singh
MBBS, MS, DNB, MNAMS
Additional Professor
Department of Anatomy
All Indian Institute of Medical Sciences (AIIMS)
Jodhpur - 342 005 (India)

SCIENTIFIC
PUBLISHERS

Published by:

Scientific Publishers (India)
5 A, New Pali Road, P.O. Box 91
Jodhpur 342 001 (India)

E-mail: info@scientificpub.com
Website: www.scientificpub.com

Branch Office
Scientific Publishers (India)
4806/24, Ansari Road, Daryaganj
New Delhi - 110 002 (India)

Print: 2017

ISBN: 978-81-7233-912-8 (Vol. 3)
978-81-7233-910-4 (Vol. 1)
978-81-7233-911-1 (Vol. 2)
978-81-7233-950-4 (Vol. 4)
978-81-7233-942-5 (Set)

Typeset by Rajesh Ojha
Printed in India

Dedicated to

My children

Vyomika Singh & Kostubh Singh

for helping me in preparing and editing this book

my wife

Dr. Ritu Singh

for positive suggestions, ideas and continuous encouragement

My teachers

Prof RK Gandhi, Prof Anil K Malhotra & Prof Ganesh Kumar

for making me believe that yesterday's young student one day will become very good teacher, person, friend, mentor and author....

My parent college

Teachers, Students & Staff of MLB Medical College, Jhansi

My students past & present

for appreciating my way of teaching - ABC of life that is - Aim, Basics & Competition ... and expecting more simpler & interesting way of Anatomy teaching from my side...

My friends & well wishers

from

All India Institute of Medical Sciences (AIIMS), Jodhpur, India

FOREWORD

Every education system is based on two important domains first-teaching/learning and preparation of subject, second important domain is - evaluation of the knowledge acquired by the candidate during first domain i.e. teaching and learning. Nowadays latest and the most scientific approach to evaluate the subjective knowledge is by multiple choice questions, i.e. MCQs. Nowadays MCQs are standard part of evaluation in MBBS and BDS Professional examinations as well as in semesters and they make about 25% to 40% of total marks at various levels during these course at all medical institutes including AIIMS across the country. More important to know is that MCQs are the only questions asked in the Medical PG Entrance exams at state, national and international level.

I appreciate the efforts by Dr. Singh in preparing this book and hope that this book `**Exam Success Review - Anatomy MCQ's for 1st Prof. MBBS & PG Entrance - by Dr. Brijendra Singh,** in three volumes - **Volume -1 Head, Neck & Brain, Volume - 2 Thorax & Upper Limb & Volume -3 Abdomen & Lower Limb** having more than 1200 MCQs in each volume will certainly help the MBBS and BDS students to secure desired merit in their exams and will also be useful for their preparations for PG Entrance examinations and help them to get the PG of their choice.

Dr. Sanjeev Misra
MBBS, MS, Mch, FRCS (England & Glasgow)
FICS, FACS (USA), FAMS
Director & CEO
AIIMS, Jodhpur, India

PREFACE

First of all I am thankful to all of my students present and past who kept me reminding continuously about the need of small, simple, handy and really concise book of anatomy subject as per their new syllabus and as per latest guidelines of **Medical Council of India**. The ultimate aim of any teaching system or educational institute is to produce the best scholars and the best professionals in the today's scenario alongwith futuristic approach that is when given a chance they must be able to exhibit their past knowledge. To verify or quantify this knowledge the student/scholar has to undergo certain set of exam. **Now-a-days the best exams are supposed to be those which are having Multiple Choice Questions ie MCQ's as integral part** because of two important reasons, First easy to conduct and uniform evaluation for all students, that is no bias, Second **MCQ's** checks memory/recall memory/ reasoning & ability to be precise in terms of reading/ understanding and speed with ability to record answers with accuracy too. The book on this subject **"Exam Success Review ANATOMY MCQ's-Volume-3, Abdomen & Lower Limb for Medical Students – MBBS-1st Prof & PG Entrance"** will be helpful as a companion for **fast revision during examination** and will certainly help them to secure full marks in the **Multiple Choice Questions** section of their examination paper. I must let you know that **MCQ's** make about 20% to 40% of total marks in the **1st Professional exam** and any student who knows the concepts and art to answer the **Multiple Choice Questions** is going to be winner not only at **MBBS** but also at various **Postgraduate Entrance Examinations** at national & state level. One shall remember that **MCQ's** are **the only questions which are asked in PG Entrance Examinations** so practice MCQ's from **1st year of MBBS** will be the best bet for any **MBBS** student for not only securing the best score in **MBBS** exams but also in **PG Entrance Examinations**. Keeping all this in mind and realizing the need of this type of systematic and authentic book on subject as well as continuous demand from various groups of students, this **MCQ** book **"Exam Success Review ANATOMY MCQ-Volume-3, Abdomen & Lower Limb for Medical Students – MBBS-1st Prof & PG Entrance"** is crafted for you all, to make your dreams of getting best marks in **MBBS** and **PG Entrance Exam** success a reality.

I will be thankful for your evaluation of morethan **1400 MCQ's** of this volume and your suggestions, feedbacks will be of very much value for making this book more useful to the students in future.

All the best for your future ventures......

Good luck & Happy reading .....

Dr. Brijendra Singh
MBBS, MS, DNB, MNAMS
Additional Professor of Anatomy
AIIMS Jodhpur India
E-mail: drbrijendrasingh@gmail.com

ACKNOWLEDGEMENT

First of all I would like to say my sincere thanks from the core of my heart to **Prof Dr. Sanjeev Misra CEO & Director of AIIMS, Jodhpur, India,** for his inspiration, unconditional support & continuous encouragement to create & complete my third book **"Exam Success Review ANATOMY MCQ's-Volume-3, Abdomen & Lower Limb for Medical Students - MBBS-1st Prof & PG Entrance"**.

I am grateful and pay my sincere regards and thanks to my anchors and motivators, Prof Sanjeev Misra Director AIIMS Jodhpur, Prof MC Mishra Director AIIMS New Delhi, Prof GK Singh Director AIIMS Patna, Prof Raj Kumar Director AIIMS Rishikesh, Prof Nitin Nagarkar Director AIIMS Raipur, Prof Sandeep Kumar Director AIIMS Bhopal, Dr. Sunil Khattri Director Rajeev Gandhi Super Speciality Hospital New Delhi, Dr. AK Bhatt, Director GNMU Greater Noida & Prof Ravi Kant Vice Chancellor King George Medical University, Lucknow.

I am also thankful to my colleagues Prof. S Ghatak, Dr. Renu Gupta, Dr. Dushyant Agrawal & Dr. Ashish Kumar Nayyar all from the department of Anatomy at AIIMS, Jodhpur for their continuous and positive criticism for making this book better and student friendly.

I am really thankful to my colleagues Prof Latika Mohan, & Prof Saurabh Varshneye from AIIMS Rishikesh, Prof DK Sharma, Dr. Vijya Kumar & Dr. Abu Siddique of AIIMS Raipur, Prof. Bertha Rathinam of AIIMS Bhopal, Prof TS Roy & Prof A Sarif, from AIIMS, New Delhi.

I am also thankful to Prof G N Quazi, Vice Chancellor of Jamia Hamdard New Delhi & Prof Raj D Mehra, Department of Anatomy, HIMSR, Jamia Hamdard New Delhi, for their support and encouragement.

I also thank my senior colleagues Prof Rani Kumar, Dean Hindu Rao Medical College Delhi, Prof. Vishram Singh & Dr. Ruchira Sethi, Santosh Medical College, Ghaziabad, Prof. Gayatri Rath, Prof. Vandana Mehta, Prof RK Suri, Prof Hitendra Kumar & Dr. Prabhat Goel of VMCC Medical College & Safdarjang Hospital, New Delhi, Prof. Veena Bharihoke, UCMS, New Delhi, Prof. Sneh Agarwal, LHMC, New Delhi & Prof Dinesh Arya from MAMC, New Delhi.

My sincere thanks to Prof. Daisy Shahni & Dr. Anjali, PGI-Chandigarh, Prof. Kanchan Kapoor, Govt Medical College Chandigarh, Prof. Patnaik Gopichand VV, Dean, MMIMSR, Mullana Ambala, for their continuous encouragement.

My thanks are due for Prof. V. Kumar, Dr. Nitya Nand & Dr. Adil ashgar of RIMSR Safai, Prof. R.K. Srivastava, Rama Medical College Kanpur, Prof A K Singh MLN Medical College, Allahabad, Dr. Pramod Kumar, Dr. Hamid Ansari of GSVM, Medical College Kanpur, Prof. Ashok Garg, Saraswati Medical College, Hapur, Prof Shobha Bhatnagar & Dr. Gyan Prakash Mishra of Carrier Medical College, Lucknow, Prof. Kamlesh Khatri, Sharda University, Greater Noida.

I would also like to say words of thanks to Prof. SL Jethani & Prof RK Rohatgi from HIMS, Dehradun, Prof DN Sinha, Prof AK Singh of GMC Haldwani, Prof. SK Jain, Teerthankar University, Moradabad, Prof. Ramesh Babu & Prof. Kuldeep singh, Muzaffarnagar Medical College, Muzaffarnagar, Prof. Archana Sharma & Dr. GL Nigam of LLRM Medical College Meerut, Prof. DR Singh, Prof. Ashok Sahai, Prof. PK Sharma, Prof. AK Srivastava, Prof. Punita Manik & Prof. Navneet Chohan from KGMU, Lucknow, Prof. MS Siddiqui of Era's Medical College, Lucknow, Prof. Biswa Bina Ray of ESIC Medical College, Bengaluru, Prof. Zora Singh & Dr. Poonam of Baba Farid University of Health Sciences Faridkot, Punjab, Prof. Rajan Singla & Dr. Gaurav Agnihotri from GMC, Amritsar, Prof. Sushma Kataria & Dr. Anoop, of SN Medical College, Jodhpur, Prof. Vasundhra Kulshrestha, SN Medical College, Agra, Prof. NK Goyal, Hind Medical College, Barabanki, Prof. Nafish Faruqi and Prof. SM Yunis of AMU, Prof. SK Pandey from IMS BHU.

I will remain thankful to all senior faculty members as well as colleagues, staff and students of AIIMS, JODHPUR for their support, encouragement & feedback given time to time.

My full regards & thanks to my beloved teachers, mentors and guide Prof RK Gandhi, Prof Mridula Kapoor, Prof SP Singh, Prof DP Singh & Prof RJ Thomas for their guidance and support. My special thanks are due for my mentors/seniors Dr. Niraj Garg & Dr. Indu GArg from Meerut.

My special thanks are due for my friends Dr. Sudhir Kumar, Dr. D.K. Sirohi & Dr. Ramkumar Ashoka for their motivation and well wishes.

My special thanks are due for Mr. Vishan Lal Ji, Librarian at MLB Medical College, and Kasif Khan Librarian at Era Medical College for assistance & valuable suggestions.

My special thanks to my family for their full support in completion of third volume of this book as well as for sacrificing their demands and time from my side which is invested in this noble work. I am thankful to my daughter Vyomika Singh and son Kostubh Singh for being patient and non-demanding as well as helping me to complete this book in many aspects. I will fail if I forget to appreciate and to say words of thanks to my best friend and wife Dr. Ritu Singh for her continuous support and every help at every small step in preparing this book & continuous encouragement which she extended at times when it was needed the most.

I am very much thankful to Mr. Tanay Sharma, Managing Director, Scientific Publishers (India), Jodhpur for timely workup editing and final printing even less than the expected time period.

I am and will remain indebted to almighty **God Lord Krishna** with folded hands for his blessings so that my third book **"Exam Success Review ANATOMY MCQ's-Volume-3, Abdomen & Lower Limb for Medical Students - MBBS-1st Prof & PG Entrance"** could become a reality and will prove to be useful for readers today, tomorrow & ever.

Thanks & All the best....

Dr. Brijendra Singh
MBBS, MS, DNB, MNAMS
Additional Professor of Anatomy
AIIMS Jodhpur India
E-mail: drbrijendrasingh@gmail.com

CONTENTS

Part - 1
Abdomen

Chapter 1

Stomach

1. Most dilated part of digestive tube is-
   (A) stomach
   (B) caecum
   (C) sigmoid colon
   (D) rectum

2. Stomach secretes hormone-
   (A) gastric acid
   (B) gastrin
   (C) intrinsic factor
   (D) all of the above

3. Capacity of stomach in adults is-
   (A) ½- 1 ltrs
   (B) 1-1½ ltrs
   (C) 1½ -2 ½ ltrs
   (D) 2-3 ltrs

4. Capacity of stomach in newborn is-
   (A) 300-500 ml
   (B) 30 -50 ml
   (C) 100 -200 ml
   (D) 500-1000 ml

5. Stomach is located in-
   (A) epigastrium & right hypochondriac region
   (B) epigastrium & right hypochondriac & umbilical region
   (C) epigastrium & left hypochondriac & umbilicus
   (D) epigastrium & left hypochondriac & right hypochondriac region

6. Volume of fundic air in empty stomach is-
   (A) 50 ml
   (B) 100ml
   (C) 200 ml
   (D) 500ml

7. Cardiac orifice of stomach is-
   (A) T 11 vertebral level
   (B) 40 cms from upper central incisor
   (C) 1 inch left to median plane behind 7th costal cartilage
   (D) all of the above

8. Pyloric orifice of stomach is-
   (A) T 11 vertebral level
   (B) T12 vertebral level
   (C) L1 vertebral level
   (D) L2 vertebral level

9. True about pyloric sphincter is-
(A) related to pre pyloric vein of Mayo
(B) bile stained after death
(C) remains open in empty stomach
(D) all of the above

10. Pylorus is related anteriorly to-
(A) caudate lobe of liver
(B) quadrate lobe of liver
(C) bare area of liver
(D) all of the above

11. Pylorus is related posteriorly to-
(A) lesser sac
(B) neck of pancreas
(C) both
(D) none of the above

12. True about lesser curvature is
(A) more fixed than greater curvature
(B) more posterior than greater curvature
(C) incisura angularis at transpyloric plane
(D) all of the above

13. Lesser curvature have anastomosis between –
(A) right & left gastroepiploic artery
(B) right & left gastric arteries
(C) both
(D) none

14. Greater curvature have anastomosis between –
(A) right & left gastroepiploic artery
(B) right & left gastric arteries
(C) both
(D) none

15. Pyloric antrum is a bulge seen at-
(A) lesser curvature
(B) greater curvature
(C) both
(D) none

16. Fundus of the stomach reaches upto-
(A) left 10th intercostal space
(B) left 8th intercostal space
(C) left 7th intercostal space
(D) left 5th intercostal space

17. Ligament attached at cardiac end is-
(A) gastro splenic ligament
(B) gastro phrenic ligament
(C) lesser omentum
(D) all of the above

18. Ligament attached at fundus of stomach is-
(A) gastro splenic ligament
(B) gastro phrenic ligament
(C) lesser omentum
(D) all of the above

19. Anterior surface of stomach is related to -
(A) greater sac
(B) diaphragm
(C) quadrate & left lobe of liver
(D) all of the above

20. Gastric triangle is on-
(A) anterior surface of stomach
(B) posterior surface of stomach
(C) posterior surface of liver
(D) posterior surface of spleen

21. Boundaries of gastric triangle are-
(A) right- inferior border of liver
(B) left – left costal margin
(C) inferior- transverse colon
(D) all of the above

22. Traube's space is –
(A) over the fundus of stomach
(B) tympanic on percussion
(C) obliterated by splenomegaly/ hepatomegaly/pleural effusion
(D) all are true

23. Traube 's space is bounded by-
(A) superiorly - inferior border of left lung
(B) right – inferior border of left lobe of liver
(C) left- lateral end of spleen
(D) all of the above

24. Viscera forming stomach bed are separated by lesser sac except-
(A) left supra renal gland
(B) spleen
(C) left crus of diaphragm
(D) splenic artery

25. Venous drainage of stomach is-
(A) right & left gastric veins -portal vein
(B) short gastric & left gastroepiploic veins- splenic vein
(C) right gastro epiploic veins-superior mesenteric veins
(D) all of the above

26. Sympathetic nerve supply to stomach comes from-
(A) T2-T10
(B) T4-T12
(C) T6-T9
(D) T6-T12

27. True about nerve of Latrjet is all except-
(A) branch from right vagus
(B) main gastric branch of anterior vagal trunk
(C) runs at lesser curvature & supply anterior surface except pylorus
(D) terminal branches supply pyloric antrum

28. Nerve of Grassi is-
(A) supplies fundus of stomach
(B) arises at gastro-esophageal junction
(C) branch from posterior vagal trunk
(D) all of the above

29. Right vagus in neck –
(A) becomes anterior vagus in abdomen
(B) becomes posterior vagus in abdomen
(C) both are true
(D) none of the above

30. Lesser omentum is attached to-
(A) lesser curvature of stomach
(B) lesser curvature of stomach & oesophagus
(C) lesser curvature of stomach & 1st part of duodenum
(D) lesser curvature of stomach , 1st part of duodenum & liver

31. Lesser omentum at lesser curvature contains –
(A) right & left gastric vessels
(B) right & left gastric vessels + gastric branches of vagus nerve
(C) right & left gastric vessels+ gastric branches of vagus nerve+ lymph nodes
(D) right gastric vessels+ gastric branches of vagus nerve

32. Free margin of lesser omentum contains-
(A) portal vein & bile duct
(B) portal vein , bile duct & hepatic artery
(C) hepatic artery, sympathetic plexus, bile duct & portal vein
(D) none of the above

33. Lesser omentum has-
(A) hepato-gastric ligament
(B) hepato-splenic ligament
(C) hepato duodenal part
(D) a & c

34. Lesser omentum develops from –
(A) anterior part of dorsal mesogastrium
(B) posterior part of ventral mesogastrium
(C) anterior part of ventral mesogastrium
(D) all of the above

35. True about greater omentum is-
(A) largest peritoneal fold – four layers
(B) 2nd & 3rd are continuous & derived from lesser sac
(C) 1st & 4th are continuous & derived from greater sac
(D) all are true

36. Contents in the space between 1st & 2nd layer of greater omentum are-
(A) left & right gastro-epiploic arteries
(B) right & left gastric artery
(C) a & b
(D) none

37. Greater omentum develops from-
(A) ventral mesogastrium
(B) dorsal mesogastrium
(C) both a & b
(D) none of the above

38. True about gastro-splenic ligament is-
(A) anterior layer is derived from greater sac
(B) posterior layer is derived from lesser sac
(C) connects fundus of stomach to upper lip of hilum of spleen
(D) all are true

39. Gastro-splenic ligament develops from-
(A) ventral mesogastrium
(B) anterior part of dorsal mesogastrium
(C) posterior part of dorsal mesogastrium
(D) none of the above

40. Contents in gastro splenic ligament are-
(A) short gastric & left gastro-epiploic arteries
(B) right & left gastric artery
(C) right gastric artery & right gastro epiploic artery
(D) none

41. True about gastro-phrenic ligament is-
(A) derived from lesser sac
(B) connects left crus of diaphragm to cardiac end of stomach
(C) contents are left gastric artery & part of left supra renal gland
(D) all of the above

42. Stomach develops in-
(A) 6th week
(B) 5th week
(C) 4th week
(D) 7th week

43. Stomach develops from-
(A) foregut
(B) midgut
(C) foregut & midgut both
(D) none of the above

44. Spleen develops from fore gut in-
(A) ventral mesogastrium
(B) dorsal mesogastrium
(C) both a & b
(D) none

45. Most distensible and dilated part of digestive tube is-
(A) stomach
(B) sigmoid colon
(C) rectum
(D) caecum

Answersheet

1. **B**	2. **B**	3. **B**	4. **B**	5. **B**	6. **A**	7. **D**	8. **C**	9. **D**	10. **B**
11. **C**	12. **D**	13. **B**	14. **A**	15. **B**	16. **D**	17. **B**	18. **A**	19. **D**	20. **A**
21. **D**	22. **D**	23. **D**	24. **B**	25. **D**	26. **C**	27. **A**	28. **D**	29. **B**	30. **D**
31. **C**	32. **C**	33. **D**	34. **B**	35. **D**	36. **A**	37. **B**	38. **D**	39. **B**	40. **A**
41. **D**	42. **C**	43. **A**	44. **B**	45. **A**					

Chapter **2**

Duodenum, Pancreas, Spleen and Liver

1. Small intestine extends from-
(A) pyloric end of stomach to appendix
(B) pyloric end of stomach to caecum
(C) pyloric end of stomach to ileo-caecal junction
(D) pyloric end of stomach to right colic flexure

2. Fixed part of small intestine is-
(A) duodenum
(B) jejunum
(C) ileum
(D) caecum

3. Part of small intestine not having mesentery is-
(A) duodenum
(B) jejunum
(C) ileum
(D) caecum

4. Length of duodenum is-
(A) 10 cms
(B) 15 cms
(C) 25 cms
(D) 40 cms

5. Length of first part of duodenum is-
(A) 5 cms
(B) 10 cms
(C) 2.5 cms
(D) 25 cms

6. Length of second part of duodenum is-
(A) 5 cms
(B) 10 cms
(C) 2.5 cms
(D) 25 cms

7. Length of third part of duodenum is-
(A) 5 cms
(B) 10 cms
(C) 2.5 cms
(D) 25 cms

8. Length of fourth part of duodenum is-
(A) 5 cms
(B) 10 cms
(C) 2.5 cms
(D) 25 cms

9. First part of duodenum is-
(A) pylorus to superior duodenal flexure
(B) directed superiorly-posteriorly & to right
(C) 5cms in length
(D) all of the above

10. First part of duodenum is related anteriorly to-
(A) quadrate lobe of liver
(B) neck of gall bladder
(C) body of gall bladder
(D) all of the above

11. First part of duodenum is –
(A) anteriorly covered with peritoneum of greater sac
(B) posteriorly covered with peritoneum
(C) not covered with peritoneum
(D) none of the above

12. Posterior surface is non peritoneal –
(A) except for part close to pylorus
(B) completely non peritoneal
(C) except for superior duodenal flexure
(D) a & c

13. Posterior surface of duodenum first part is related to-
(A) portal vein
(B) bile duct & gastroduodenal artery
(C) inferior vena cava
(D) all of the above

14. Superior border/surface of first part of duodenum is-
(A) attachment of free margin of lesser omentum
(B) forms floor of epiploic foramen
(C) hepatic artery
(D) all of the above

15. End arteries supply to-
(A) 1st part of duodenum
(B) 2nd part of duodenum
(C) 3rd part of duodenum
(D) 4th part of duodenum

16. Arterial supply of first part of duodenum is-
(A) supra duodenal branch of gastroduodenal artery
(B) retroduodenal branch of gastroduodenal artery
(C) infraduodenal branch of right gastro epiploic artery
(D) all of the above

17. Artery of Wilkie which is an end artery is-
(A) supra duodenal branch of gastroduodenal artery
(B) retroduodenal branch of gastroduodenal artery
(C) infraduodenal branch of right gastro epiploic artery
(D) all of the above

18. Duodenal cap is formed by-
(A) 1st part of duodenum
(B) 2nd part of duodenum
(C) 3rd part of duodenum
(D) 4th part of duodenum

19. Most movable part of duodenum is -
(A) 1st part of duodenum
(B) 2nd part of duodenum
(C) 3rd part of duodenum
(D) 4th part of duodenum

20. First part of duodenum lies against-
(A) L1
(B) L2
(C) L3
(D) L4

21. Second part of duodenum is-
(A) 8-10 cms in length
(B) vertical part
(C) extends –from- L1 to L3 vertebrae
(D) all of the above

22. Anterior relations of 2nd part of duodenum are-
(A) right lobe of liver
(B) transverse colon
(C) coils of jejunum
(D) all of the above

23. Non peritoneal anterior relations of 2nd part of duodenum is -
(A) right lobe of liver
(B) transverse colon
(C) coils of jejunum
(D) all of the above

24. Posterior relations of 2nd part of duodenum are-
(A) hilum of right kidney
(B) right psoas major muscle
(C) right border of inferior vena cava
(D) all of the above

25. Medial relations of 2nd part of duodenum are-
(A) head of pancreas
(B) bile & main pancreatic duct
(C) superior & inferior pancreticoduodenal arteries
(D) all of the above

26. Lateral relations of 2nd part of duodenum are-
(A) head of pancreas
(B) right colic flexure
(C) transverse colon
(D) right psoas major muscle

27. Accessory pancreatic duct opens-
(A) minor duodenal papilla with major duodenal papilla
(B) minor duodenal papilla 2 cms distal to major duodenal papilla
(C) minor duodenal papilla 2 cms proximal to major duodenal papilla
(D) all of the above

28. Major duodenal papilla –
(A) present in 2nd part of duodenum
(B) opens on postero-medial surface
(C) both pancreatic & bile duct open on it
(D) all of the above

29. Major duodenal papilla is located by -
(A) plica longitudenalis
(B) plica circularis
(C) plica semicircularis
(D) all of the above

30. Monk hood at major duodenal papilla is formed by -
(A) plica longitudenalis
(B) plica circularis
(C) plica semicircularis
(D) all of the above

31. True about third part of duodenum –
(A) 10 cms long horizontal part
(B) rests over abdominal aorta & inferior vena cava
(C) anterior to L3 vertebra
(D) all of the above

32. Anterior relations of 3rd part of duodenum –
(A) covered with peritoneum
(B) crossed by root of mesentery
(C) crossed by superior mesenteric artery
(D) all are true

33. Posterior relations of 3rd part of duodenum are all except –
(A) inferior vena cava
(B) inferior mesenteric artery
(C) superior mesenteric artery
(D) abdominal aorta

34. Posterior relations of 3rd part of duodenum are –
(A) right ureter
(B) right gonadal vessels
(C) right psoas major muscle
(D) all are true

35. Superior relations of 3rd part of duodenum is –
(A) inferior vena cava
(B) superior mesenteric artery
(C) head of pancreas & inferior pancretico-duodenal artery
(D) abdominal aorta

36. True about fourth part of duodenum is-
(A) 5 cms in length
(B) opposite to L3
(C) opposite to L2
(D) anterior to Inferior vena cava

37. Shortest part of duodenum is
(A) 1st part
(B) 2nd part
(C) 3rd part
(D) 4th part

38. Longest part of duodenum is
(A) 1st part
(B) 2nd part
(C) 3rd part
(D) 4th part

39. Longest part of duodenum is
(A) upper part
(B) vertical part
(C) horizontal part
(D) ascending part

40. Fourth part of duodenum extends from–
(A) front of aorta to duodeno-jejunal flexure
(B) front of inferior vena cava to duodeno-jejunal flexure
(C) duodeno-duodenal flexure to duodeno-jejunal flexure
(D) none of the above

41. Anterior relations of 4th part of duodenum is-
(A) left renal vessels
(B) stomach
(C) inferior mesenteric vein
(D) all of the above

42. Anterior relations of 4th part of duodenum is-
(A) transverse colon
(B) stomach
(C) transverse mesocolon
(D) all of the above

43. Superior relations of 4th part of duodenum –
(A) head of pancreas
(B) body of pancreas
(C) tail of pancreas
(D) all of the above

44. Left relations of 4th part of duodenum are-
(A) left kidney
(B) left ureter
(C) both
(D) none

45. Right relations of 4th part of duodenum are-
(A) right kidney
(B) right suprarenal
(C) uncinate process of pancreas
(D) head of pancreas

46. Posterior relations of 4th part of duodenum are-
(A) left crus of diaphragm
(B) left renal vessels
(C) left gonadal vessels
(D) all of the above

47. True about suspensory muscle of Treitz-
(A) arises from right crus of diaphragm
(B) reaches to duodeno-jejunal flexure
(C) fibro muscular band
(D) all of the above

48. True about suspensory muscle of Treitz-
(A) upper 1/3 striated muscle
(B) middle 1/3 elastic tissue
(C) lower 1/3 unstriated muscle
(D) all of the above

49. Brunner's gland are seen in-
(A) stomach
(B) duodenum
(C) ileum
(D) jejunum

50. Brunner's glands are present in –
(A) mucosal layer
(B) sub mucosal layer
(C) serosal layer
(D) muscularis interna

51. Nerve supply of duodenum comes from-
(A) coeliac plexus
(B) superior mesenteric plexus
(C) vagus nerves
(D) all of the above

52. Sympathetic nerves are derived from-
(A) T2-T8
(B) T4-T8 part of duodenum
(C) T6-T9
(D) T8-T12

53. Annular pancreas commonly involves-
(A) 1st part of duodenum
(B) 2nd part of duodenum
(C) 3rd part of duodenum
(D) 4th part of duodenum

54. Part of duodenum most vulnerable to external injury is -
(A) 1st part of duodenum
(B) 2nd part of duodenum
(C) 3rd part of duodenum
(D) 4th part of duodenum

55. Part of duodenum related to paraduodenal recess-
(A) 1st part of duodenum
(B) 2nd part of duodenum
(C) 3rd part of duodenum
(D) 4th part of duodenum

56. True about meckel's diverticulum is-
(A) blind pouch arises from anti mesenteric border of ileum
(B) 2 feet proximal to ileo caecal junction
(C) 2 inches long & present in 2% of population
(D) all are true

57. Meckel's diverticulum is remnant of-
(A) vitello intestinal duct
(B) urachus
(C) para mesonephric duct
(D) all of the above

58. Vitello intestinal duct connects –
(A) fore gut to extra embryonic part of yolk sac
(B) mid gut to extra embryonic part of yolk sac
(C) hind gut to extra embryonic part of yolk sac
(D) mid gut to intra embryonic part of yolk sac

59. Length of small intestine in living is-
(A) 6 mtrs
(B) 7 mtrs
(C) 8 mtrs
(D) 9mtrs

60. M cells are seen –
(A) muscle cells
(B) epithelial cells covering payer's patches
(C) mucosal cells in duodenum
(D) all of the above

61. True about pancreas is all except-
(A) lies retroperitoneally
(B) separated from stomach by lesser sac
(C) separated from stomach by greater sac
(D) both endo & exocrine gland

62. True about pancreas is all except-
(A) present in epigastrium
(B) present in left hypochondrium
(C) forms stomach bed separated by greater sac
(D) forms stomach bed separated by lesser sac

63. Neck of the pancreas is lying-
(A) anterior to Inferior Vena Cava
(B) anterior to portal vein
(C) posterior to portal vein
(D) anterior to aorta

64. Part of pancreas triangular on cross section is-
(A) head
(B) neck
(C) body
(D) tail

65. Part of pancreas anterior to abdominal aorta & left kidney is-
(A) head
(B) neck
(C) body
(D) tail

66. Head of pancreas lies opposite to-
(A) T12-L1 vertebrae
(B) L1-L2 vertebrae
(C) L1 vertebra
(D) L2 vertebra

67. Head and neck of pancreas anteriorly are demarcated by-
(A) superior mesenteric artery
(B) portal vein
(C) gastro duodenal artery
(D) all of the above

68. All are related to anterior surface of head of pancreas except-
(A) transverse colon
(B) inferior vena cava
(C) coils of jejunum
(D) superior mesenteric artery

69. Posterior relations of head of pancreas–
(A) inferior vena cava
(B) right renal vein
(C) left renal vein
(D) all if the above

70. Posterior relations of head of pancreas-
(A) right crus of diaphragm
(B) right middle supra renal artery
(C) right gonadal artery
(D) all of the above

71. Structure lodged between second part of duodenum and head of pancreas posteriorly –
(A) inferior vena cava
(B) bile duct
(C) right renal vein
(D) all of the above

72. True about relations of uncinated process of pancreas is-
(A) abdominal aorta posteriorly
(B) anteriorly superior mesenteric vessels
(C) superiorly left renal vein
(D) all of the above

73. Neck of pancreas is related to all except-
(A) anteriorly pylorus of stomach
(B) superior mesenteric vein posteriorly
(C) portal vein posteriorly
(D) inferior vena cava posteriorly

74. All are related to antero-inferior surface of pancreas except-
(A) lesser sac & stomach
(B) greater sac & duodeno-jejunal junction
(C) left colic flexure
(D) coils of jejunum

75. Posterior relations of body of pancreas are –
(A) left crus of diaphragm
(B) left supra renal gland
(C) abdominal aorta
(D) all of the above

76. Posterior relations of body of pancreas are-
(A) left ureter
(B) left renal vessels
(C) splenic vein
(D) all of the above

77. All are true for superior border of pancreas except-
(A) splenic vein
(B) tuber omentale
(C) hepatic artery
(D) splenic artery

78. Root of transverse mesocolon is attached to-
(A) superior border
(B) anterior border
(C) inferior border
(D) all of the above

79. Most mobile part of pancreas is-
(A) head
(B) neck
(C) body
(D) tail

80. Tail of the pancreas is lying opposite to-
(A) T11 vertebra
(B) T12 vertebra
(C) L1 vertebra
(D) L2 vertebra

81. Main pancreatic duct is called-
(A) duct of Santorini
(B) duct of Wirsung
(C) duct of Stenson
(D) duct of Rivinus

82. Accessory pancreatic duct is called-
(A) duct of Santorini
(B) duct of Wirsung
(C) duct of Stenson
(D) duct of Rivinus

83. Herring bone pattern is seen in-
(A) developing bone
(B) pancreatic duct
(C) both a & b
(D) none of the above

84. Duct of Santorini receives secretions from-
(A) head of pancreas
(B) uncinate process
(C) body of pancreas
(D) all of the above

85. Arterial supply of pancreas is from-
(A) splenic artery
(B) superior pancreatico-duodenal artery
(C) inferior pancreatico-duodenal artery
(D) all of the above

86. Venous drainage of pancreas –
(A) superior mesenteric vein
(B) splenic vein
(C) portal vein
(D) all of the above

87. Accessory pancreatic tissue may be seen in-
(A) stomach
(B) duodenum
(C) spleen
(D) all of the above

88. Accessory pancreatic tissue is most commonly seen in-
(A) stomach
(B) duodenum
(C) spleen
(D) greater omentum

89. Main blood supply of pancreas is from-
(A) splenic artery
(B) superior pancreatico-duodenal artery
(C) inferior pancreatico-duodenal artery
(D) all of the above

90. Most movable part of duodenum is-
(A) first part
(B) second part
(C) third part
(D) fourth part

91. Most involved part of duodenum in peptic ulcers is-
(A) first part
(B) second part
(C) third part
(D) fourth part

92. Most commonly injured part of duodenum in external trauma is-
(A) first part
(B) second part
(C) third part
(D) fourth part

93. Most of islets of Langerhans are seen in-
(A) head of pancreas
(B) body of pancreas
(C) tail of pancreas
(D) no such distribution

94. Largest gland of the body is-
(A) pancreas
(B) liver
(C) large intestine
(D) none of the above

95. Functions of liver are –
(A) synthesis of proteins
(B) haemopoisis
(C) storage of glycogen
(D) all of the above

96. In midline upper border of liver lies at-
(A) level of xiphisternal joint
(B) level of T12
(C) trans pyloric level
(D) none of the above

97. In midline upper border of liver lies at-
(A) level of xiphisternal joint
(B) level of T12
(C) trans pyloric level
(D) none of the above

98. Weight of the liver in adults is-
(A) 1/18th of body weight
(B) 1/30th of body weight
(C) 1/40th of body weight
(D) none of the above

99. Weight of the liver in neonates is-
(A) 1/18th of body weight
(B) 1/30th of body weight
(C) 1/40th of body weight
(D) none of the above

100. Only well defined border of liver is –
(A) anterior border
(B) superior border
(C) inferior border
(D) posterior border

101. Areas of liver not covered by peritoneum are-
(A) fossa for inferior vena cava
(B) fossa for gall bladder
(C) porta hepatis
(D) all of the above

102. All are false ligaments of liver except-
(A) falciform ligament
(B) right triangular ligament
(C) ligamentum venosum
(D) coronary ligament

103. All are false ligaments of liver except-
(A) falciform ligament
(B) left triangular ligament
(C) ligamentum teres hepatica
(D) coronary ligament

104. Right lateral surface of liver extends from-
(A) 5 to 10 ribs in mid axillary line
(B) 6 to 10 ribs in mid axillary line
(C) 7 to 11 ribs in mid axillary line
(D) 7 to 12 ribs in mid axillary line

105. Liver is kept in its position because of-
(A) hepatic veins
(B) intra abdominal pressure
(C) peritoneal ligaments
(D) all of the above

106. Cystohepatic angle is an angle between-
(A) right & left hepatic ducts
(B) common hepatic duct & cystic duct
(C) common bile duct & cystic duct
(D) none of the above

107. Part of gall bladder which is completely intraperitoneal is-
(A) neck of gall bladder
(B) body of gall bladder
(C) fundus of gall bladder
(D) whole gall bladder

108. Hartmann's pouch is seen in –
(A) neck of gall bladder
(B) body of gall bladder
(C) fundus of gall bladder
(D) common bile duct of gall bladder

109. First part of duodenum is related to-
(A) neck of gall bladder
(B) body of gall bladder
(C) fundus of gall bladder
(D) common bile duct of gall bladder

110. Nerve supply of gall bladder is –
(A) right phrenic nerve
(B) vagus nerve
(C) T7 –T9 sympathetic fibers
(D) all of the above

111. Pain in gall bladder diseases is referred to-
(A) right shoulder tip
(B) inferior angle of scapula
(C) stomach
(D) all of the above

112. Valve of HIESTER is seen in –
(A) cystic duct
(B) common bile duct
(C) neck of gall bladder
(D) none of the above

113. All form the boundaries of Calot's triangle except-
(A) inferior border of liver
(B) cystic duct on right side
(C) common bile duct on left side
(D) common hepatic duct on left side

114. Contents of Calot's triangle are-
(A) right hepatic artery
(B) cystic artery
(C) lymph node of Lund
(D) all of the above

115. Only part of liver covered by peritoneum of lesser sac is-
(A) quadrate lobe
(B) caudate lobe
(C) left lobe
(D) all of the above

Answersheet

1. **C**	2. **A**	3. **A**	4. **C**	5. **A**	6. **B**	7. **B**	8. **C**	9. **D**	10. **D**
11. **A**	12. **A**	13. **D**	14. **D**	15. **A**	16. **D**	17. **A**	18. **A**	19. **A**	20. **A**
21. **D**	22. **D**	23. **B**	24. **D**	25. **D**	26. **B**	27. **C**	28. **D**	29. **D**	30. **C**
31. **D**	32. **D**	33. **C**	34. **D**	35. **C**	36. **C**	37. **D**	38. **C**	39. **C**	40. **A**
41. **B**	42. **D**	43. **B**	44. **C**	45. **C**	46. **D**	47. **D**	48. **D**	49. **B**	50. **B**
51. **D**	52. **C**	53. **B**	54. **C**	55. **D**	56. **D**	57. **A**	58. **B**	59. **A**	60. **B**
61. **C**	62. **C**	63. **B**	64. **C**	65. **C**	66. **B**	67. **C**	68. **B**	69. **D**	70. **D**
71. **B**	72. **D**	73. **D**	74. **A**	75. **D**	76. **D**	77. **A**	78. **B**	79. **D**	80. **B**
81. **B**	82. **A**	83. **B**	84. **B**	85. **D**	86. **D**	87. **D**	88. **B**	89. **A**	90. **A**
91. **A**	92. **C**	93. **C**	94. **B**	95. **D**	96. **A**	97. **C**	98. **C**	99. **A**	100. **C**
101. **D**	102. **C**	103. **C**	104. **C**	105. **D**	106. **B**	107. **C**	108. **A**	109. **A**	110. **D**
111. **D**	112. **A**	113. **C**	114. **D**	115. **B**					

Chapter 3

Large Intestine, Rectum and Anal canal

1. True about mesentery is -
   (A) broad fan shaped fold of peritoneum
   (B) suspends jejunum & ileum
   (C) derived from greater sac
   (D) all are true

2. Root of mesentery is-
   (A) vertebral border or called as root
   (B) extends from left side of L2 to right sacro iliac joint
   (C) extends from duodeno-jejunal flexure to ileo-caecal junction
   (D) all of the above

3. Part of duodenum crossed by root of mesentery is -
   (A) 1st part of duodenum
   (B) 2nd part of duodenum
   (C) 3rd part of duodenum
   (D) 4th part of duodenum

4. Blood vessels crossed by root of mesentery are –
   (A) abdominal aorta
   (B) inferior vena cava
   (C) right gonadal vessels
   (D) all of the above

5. Root of mesentery crosses –
   (A) right sacro iliac joint
   (B) left sacro iliac joint
   (C) right side of L2
   (D) none of the above

6. Structures crossed by root of mesentery are –
   (A) right psoas major
   (B) right ureter
   (C) right genito-femoral nerve
   (D) all of the above

7. Free border of mesentery is about-
   (A) 15 feet long
   (B) 18 feet long
   (C) 20 feet long
   (D) 30 feet long

8. Contents of mesentery are-
   (A) jejunum & ileum
   (B) superior mesenteric vessels
   (C) mesenteric lymph nodes & fat
   (D) all of the above

9. Occasionally following may be contents of mesentery-
(A) tip of vermiform appendix
(B) suspensory muscle of duodenum
(C) accessory supra renal tissue
(D) all of the above

10. Characteristic features of large intestine are-
(A) taeniae coli
(B) sacculation/haustrations
(C) appendices coli
(D) all of the above

11. Taeniae coli are characteristic of large intestine are absent in-
(A) transverse colon
(B) caecum
(C) appendix
(D) sigmoid colon

12. Taeniae coli are characteristic of large intestine are absent in-
(A) transverse colon
(B) caecum
(C) rectum
(D) sigmoid colon

13. Appendices epiploicae are peritoneal pouches absent in –
(A) caecum
(B) appendix
(C) rectum
(D) all of the above

14. Faeces are generally stored in-
(A) transverse colon
(B) sigmoid colon
(C) rectum
(D) all of the above

15. Length of caecum is-
(A) 6 cm
(B) 15 cm
(C) 45 cm
(D) 25 cm

16. Length of ascending colon is-
(A) 6 cm
(B) 15 cm
(C) 45 cm
(D) 25 cm

17. Length of transverse colon is-
(A) 6 cm
(B) 15 cm
(C) 45 cm
(D) 25 cm

18. Length of descending colon is-
(A) 6 cm
(B) 15 cm
(C) 45 cm
(D) 25 cm

19. Length of sigmoid colon is-
(A) 6 cm
(B) 15 cm
(C) 40 cm
(D) 25 cm

20. Length of rectum is-
(A) 6 cm
(B) 12 cm
(C) 45 cm
(D) 25 cm

21. Length of anal canal is-
(A) 6 cm
(B) 3.8 cm
(C) 45 cm
(D) 2.5 cm

22. True about caecum is-
(A) length is 6 cms
(B) width is 7 cms
(C) is retro peritoneal
(D) all of the above

23. Most common type of caecum is-
(A) foetal type
(B) infantile type
(C) adult type
(D) exaggerated type

24. Least common type of caecum is-
(A) foetal type
(B) infantile type
(C) adult type
(D) exaggerated type

25. In foetal type of caecum true is-
(A) conical in shape
(B) appendix arises from apex
(C) seen in 2% of cases
(D) all of the above

26. In infantile type of caecum true is-
(A) quadrate in shape
(B) appendix arises from apex
(C) appendix is attached to depressed bottom
(D) a & b both
(E) a & c both

27. In exaggerated type of caecum true is-
(A) conical in shape
(B) right saccule hugely enlarges
(C) left saccule hugely enlarged
(D) b & c both

28. Caecum may be seen in –
(A) left iliac fossa
(B) umbilical region
(C) right iliac fossa
(D) sub hepatic
(E) all of the above

29. Posterior relations of caecum are-
(A) right ilio-psoas
(B) femoral nerve
(C) lateral femoral cutaneous nerve
(D) all of the above

30. Caecum continues as ascending colon at the-
(A) trans pyloric level
(B) trans tubercular plane
(C) intercristal plane
(D) umbilical level

31. Nerve supply of caecum is-
(A) sympathetic T10 –L1
(B) superior mesenteric plexus
(C) vagus
(D) all of the above

32. Lymphatic drainage of caecum is –
(A) ilio colic lymph nodes
(B) superior mesenteric group
(C) pre aortic lymph nodes
(D) all of the above

33. True about the blood supply of caecum is-
(A) anterior & posterior caecal arteries branches of ileo colic artery
(B) vein drain into ileo colic vein
(C) vein drain into superior mesenteric vein & portal vein
(D) all of the above

34. True about ileo caecal valve is-
(A) 2.5 cms in transverse plane
(B) seen at postero medial wall
(C) formed by reduplication of mucosal membrane
(D) all of the above

35. Valve of Gerlach is seen in-
(A) ileo-caecal valve
(B) appendicular orifice
(C) ileo-colic valve
(D) all of the above

36. Appendix is part of large intestine and-

(A) have taeniae coli, sacculation & appendices epiploicae

(B) have taeniae coli, sacculation & but not appendices epiploicae

(C) do not have taeniae coli, sacculation & appendices epiploicae

(D) have taeniae coli, but no sacculation & appendices epiploicae

37. Commonest position of appendix is-

(A) sub caecal

(B) retro caecal/colic

(C) pelvic type

(D) para ileal

38. Commonest position of appendix is-

(A) sub caecal

(B) retro caecal/colic

(C) pelvic type

(D) para ileal

39. Appendicular artery is-

(A) branch of inferior division of ileo colic artery

(B) is an end artery

(C) both a & b

(D) none of the above

40. Abdominal tonsil is the name given to-

(A) Payer's patches in small intestine

(B) lymph follicles in appendix

(C) lymph follicles of caecum

(D) all of the above

41. Hiatus muscularis are seen in –

(A) caecum

(B) appendix

(C) both caecum & appendix

(D) none of the above

42. Villi are absent in-

(A) appendix

(B) caecum

(C) both a & b

(D) none

43. Posterior relations of ascending colon are-

(A) right ilio –inguinal nerve

(B) right ilio-hypogastric nerve

(C) right sub costal nerve

(D) all of the above

44. Posterior relations of ascending colon are-

(A) 4th right lumbar artery

(B) sub costal artery

(C) lower pole of right kidney

(D) all of the above

45. Transverse colon right 2/3rd is supplied by-

(A) right colic artery branch of middle colic artery

(B) left colic artery branch of middle colic artery

(C) left colic artery branch of inferior mesenteric artery

(D) a & b both

(E) all of the above

46. Transverse colon left 1/3rd is supplied by-

(A) right colic artery branch of middle colic artery

(B) left colic artery branch of middle colic artery

(C) left colic artery branch of inferior mesenteric artery

(D) all of the above

47. Transverse colon right is supplied by-
(A) right colic artery branch of middle colic artery
(B) left colic artery branch of middle colic artery
(C) left colic artery branch of inferior mesenteric artery
(D) all of the above

48. Lymphatic drainage from right 2/3rd of transverse colon is-
(A) coeliac group
(B) superior mesenteric group
(C) inferior mesenteric group
(D) all of the above

49. Lymphatic drainage from left 1/3rd of transverse colon is-
(A) coeliac group
(B) superior mesenteric group
(C) inferior mesenteric group
(D) all of the above

50. Lymphatic drainage from transverse colon is-
(A) coeliac group
(B) superior mesenteric group
(C) inferior mesenteric group
(D) b & c both
(E) all of the above

51. Nerve supply of right 2/3rd of transverse colon is -
(A) sympathetic T12 –L1
(B) vagus nerve
(C) sympathetic L1-L2
(D) a & b both
(E) b & c both

52. Nerve supply of left 1/3rd of transverse colon is -
(A) sympathetic T12 –L1 & vagus nerve
(B) sympathetic L1-L2
(C) pelvic splanchnic nerves - S2,S3,S4
(D) b & c both

53. Nerve supply of transverse colon is –
(A) sympathetic T12 –L1 & vagus nerve
(B) sympathetic L1-L2
(C) pelvic splanchnic nerves - S2,S3,S4
(D) all of the above

54. Layers of transverse mesocolon in Adults are derived from-
(A) upper layer from lesser sac & lower layer from greater sac
(B) upper layer from greater sac & lower layer from lesser sac
(C) both layers from lesser sac
(D) both layers from greater sac

55. Layers of transverse mesocolon in early foetal life are derived from-
(A) upper layer from lesser sac & lower layer from greater sac
(B) upper layer from greater sac & lower layer from lesser sac
(C) both layers from lesser sac
(D) both layers from greater sac

56. Nerve supply of sigmoid colon is from-
(A) vagus
(B) superior hypo gastric plexus
(C) pelvic splanchnic nerves
(D) b & c both
(E) all of the above

57. Blood supply of sigmoid colon-
(A) 3 to 4 sigmoidal arteries from superior mesenteric artery & superior rectal artery
(B) 3 to 4 sigmoidal arteries from inferior mesenteric artery & superior rectal artery
(C) sigmoidal arteries from superior& inferior mesenteric arteries both
(D) none of the above

58. Rectum is part of large gut-
(A) have taeniae coli, sacculations & appendices epiploicae
(B) have taeniae coli, sacculations but no appendices epiploicae
(C) have taeniae coli, but no sacculations & appendices epiploicae
(D) have no taeniae coli, sacculations & appendices epiploicae

59. Rectum begins as continuation sigmoid colon at-
(A) S1 Vertebra
(B) S2 Vertebra
(C) S3 Vertebra
(D) S4 Vertebra

60. Anorectal junction in males corresponds to –
(A) apex of urinary bladder
(B) apex of prostate
(C) base of urinary bladder
(D) all of the above

61. Perineal curvature of rectum is-
(A) concave anteriorly & caused by puborectal sling of levator ani
(B) concave anteriorly & caused by pubovesicalis sling of levator ani
(C) convex anteriorly & caused by puborectal sling of levator ani
(D) convex anteriorly & caused by pubosacralis sling of levator ani

62. True about lateral curvature of rectum is –
(A) upper curvature is convex and to right
(B) upper curvature is convex and to left
(C) lower curvature is convex and to left
(D) middle curvature is convex and to right

63. True about lateral curvature of rectum is –
(A) upper curvature is convex and to left
(B) middle curvature is convex and to left
(C) lower curvature is convex and to left
(D) middle curvature is convex and to right

64. True about lateral curvature of rectum is –
(A) lower curvature is convex to left
(B) upper curvature is convex and to left
(C) lower curvature is convex and to right
(D) middle curvature is convex and to right

65. Most prominent curvature of the rectum is-
(A) upper curve
(B) middle curve
(C) lower curve
(D) all are same

66. Upper curvature of rectum is convex to right and located at-
(A) tip of coccyx
(B) sacrococcygeal junction
(C) junction of S3/S4
(D) none of the above

67. Middle curvature of rectum is convex to left and located at-
(A) tip of coccyx
(B) sacrococcygeal junction
(C) junction of S3/S4
(D) none of the above

68. Lower curvature of rectum is convex to right and located at-
(A) tip of coccyx
(B) sacrococcygeal junction
(C) junction of S3/S4
(D) none of the above

69. Non peritoneal surface of rectum is-
(A) anterior
(B) lateral
(C) posterior
(D) none of the above

70. Anterior surface of rectum is covered with peritoneum except-
(A) upper 1/3rd
(B) middle 1/3rd
(C) lower 1/3rd
(D) upper 1/2

71. Peritoneal relations of anterior surface of rectum is-
(A) base of urinary bladder
(B) seminal vesicles
(C) sigmoid colon
(D) ampulla of vas deferens

72. Non-peritoneal relations of anterior surface of rectum in males is-
(A) base of urinary bladder
(B) posterior surface of prostate
(C) seminal vesicles & ampulla of vas deferens
(D) all of the above

73. Non-peritoneal relations of anterior surface of rectum in females is-
(A) base of urinary bladder
(B) posterior surface of prostate
(C) vagina
(D) a & b both

74. Fascia of Denonvillier is –
(A) modified recto-vesical pouch
(B) present on anterior surface of rectum in males
(C) separates anteriorly urogenital organs in male
(D) all of the above

75. Fascia of Waldeyer is related to rectum-
(A) anteriorly
(B) laterally
(C) posteriorly
(D) all around

76. Rectum is related in midline posteriorly to all except-
(A) ganglion impar
(B) median sacral vessels
(C) upper three pieces of sacrum
(D) lower three pieces of sacrum

77. Rectum is related in midline posteriorly to all except-
(A) superior rectal vessels
(B) anococcygeal raphe
(C) levator ani
(D) lower three pieces of sacrum & coccyx

78. Muscles related laterally to rectum are–
(A) piriformis
(B) levator ani
(C) coccygeus
(D) all of the above

79. Lateral ligaments of rectum contains-
(A) superior rectal vessels
(B) middle rectal vessels
(C) inferior rectal vessels
(D) all of the above

80. Para rectal fossae are laterally related to rectum in-
(A) upper 1/3
(B) middle 1/3
(C) lower 1/3
(D) c & d both

81. Ischio rectal fossae are laterally related to rectum in-
(A) upper 1/3
(B) middle 1/3
(C) lower 1/3
(D) c & d both

82. Pelvi rectal space are laterally related to rectum in-
(A) upper 1/3
(B) middle 1/3
(C) lower 1/3
(D) c & d both

83. Houston valves are seen in –
(A) anal canal
(B) rectum
(C) sigmoid colon
(D) all of the above

84. Houston valves are-
(A) 2 in number
(B) 3 in number
(C) 4 in number
(D) number is not fixed

85. True about Houston valve is-
(A) formed by reduplication of mucosa
(B) horizontal in direction
(C) circular muscle of rectum is present
(D) all of the above

86. First valve of Houston is located at-
(A) recto-sigmoid junction
(B) at the S3 vertebral level
(C) about 12 to 14 cms from anus
(D) all of the above

87. Most constant among rectal valves is-
(A) first
(B) second
(C) third
(D) fourth

88. Nelaton's sphincter is-
(A) complete circular third rectal valve
(B) at the S5 level
(C) about 2 inches above the anus
(D) all are true

89. Upper part of rectum above third rectal valve-
(A) pre- allantois part of hind gut
(B) post – allantois part of hind gut
(C) mid gut
(D) none of the above

90. Principal artery of rectum is-
(A) superior rectal artery
(B) middle rectal artery
(C) inferior rectal artery
(D) none of the above

91. Superior rectal artery is a branch of –
(A) internal pudendal artery
(B) internal iliac artery
(C) inferior mesenteric artery
(D) none of the above

92. Middle rectal artery is a branch of –
(A) internal pudendal artery
(B) internal iliac artery
(C) inferior mesenteric artery
(D) none of the above

93. Inferior rectal artery is a branch of –
(A) internal pudendal artery
(B) internal iliac artery
(C) inferior mesenteric artery
(D) none of the above

94. Venous drainage of rectum is through-
(A) superior rectal vein
(B) middle rectal vein
(C) inferior rectal vein
(D) all of the above

95. Superior rectal vein drains into-
(A) inferior mesenteric vein
(B) internal iliac vein
(C) internal pudendal vein
(D) all of the above

96. Inferior rectal vein drains into-
(A) inferior mesenteric vein
(B) internal iliac vein
(C) internal pudendal vein
(D) all of the above

97. Middle rectal vein drains into-
(A) inferior mesenteric vein
(B) internal iliac vein
(C) internal pudendal vein
(D) all of the above

98. Rectal vein draining into systemic veins –
(A) superior rectal vein
(B) superior & middle rectal veins
(C) middle & inferior rectal veins
(D) none of the above

99. Rectal vein draining into portal system of veins –
(A) superior rectal vein
(B) superior & middle rectal veins
(C) middle & inferior rectal veins
(D) none of the above

100. Internal hemorrhoids are drained into-
(A) superior rectal veins
(B) middle rectal vein
(C) inferior rectal vein
(D) all of the above

101. External hemorrhoids are drained into-
(A) superior rectal veins
(B) middle rectal vein
(C) inferior rectal vein
(D) all of the above

102. True about internal hemorrhoids is-
(A) located above Hilton's line
(B) around internal anal sphincter
(C) continues into superior rectal vein
(D) all of the above

103. True about external hemorrhoids is-
(A) located below Hilton's line
(B) subcutaneous & around external anal sphincter
(C) continues into inferior rectal vein
(D) all of the above

104. Primary internal piles are located on following positions except-
(A) 2 o clock position
(B) 3 o clock position
(C) 7 o clock position
(D) 11 o clock position

105. Primary internal piles are located on following positions except-
(A) left lateral position
(B) right lateral position
(C) right anterior position
(D) right posterior position

106. Nerve supply of rectum is-
(A) sympathetic fibers from L1 L2
(B) parasympathetic fibers from S2S3S4
(C) both a & b
(D) none of the above

107. Length of anal canal is-
(A) 2.8 cms
(B) 3.8 cms
(C) 4.8 cms
(D) 5.8 cms

108. Columns of Morgagni are seen in-
(A) rectum
(B) upper part of anal canal
(C) lower part of anal canal
(D) recto-anal junction

109. Columns of Morgagni are -
(A) permanent longitudinal mucous folds
(B) 6-10 in number
(C) prominent in children
(D) all of the above

110. Anal valves located at the junction of upper and middle part –
(A) upper surface is lined by columnar epithelium
(B) above dentate line
(C) above the pectinate line
(D) all of the above

111. All are features of upper part of anal canal except-
(A) columns of Morgagni
(B) Valves of Ball
(C) Hilton's line
(D) anal glands & sinuses

112. Area of Pecten of anal canal is-
(A) upper 15 mm
(B) middle 15 mm
(C) lower 8 mm
(D) none of the above

113. True about Area of Pecten of anal canal is all except-
(A) between pectinate & Hilton's line
(B) sweat & sebaceous glands are present
(C) lined by non-keratinized stratified squamous epithelium
(D) middle 15 mm of anal canal

114. True about pectinate line of anal canal is all except-
(A) forms muco-cutaneous junction of anal canal
(B) corresponds with anal valves of Ball
(C) situated at the mid of external anal sphincter
(D) situated at the mid of internal anal sphincter

115. True about the area of anal canal superior to pectinate line is all except-
(A) develops from endoderm
(B) supplied by superior rectal artery
(C) drains into systemic veins
(D) drains into portal vein

116. True about the area of anal canal inferior to pectinate line is all except-
(A) develops from ectoderm
(B) supplied by inferior rectal artery
(C) drains into systemic veins
(D) drains into portal vein

117. Nerve supply of anal canal is-
(A) L1L2 through superior hypo gastric nerves
(B) S2S3S4 through pelvic splanchnic nerves
(C) inferior rectal nerves
(D) all of the above

118. Lymphatic drainage of anal canal is to-
(A) internal iliac nodes
(B) horizontal group of superficial inguinal nodes
(C) both A & B
(D) none of the above

119. Anal canal develops from-
(A) endodermal cloaca
(B) ectodermal proctodeum
(C) A & B both
(D) none of the above

120. True about internal anal sphincter is-
(A) involuntary
(B) formed by circular muscle
(C) in upper 1/3 of anal canal
(D) all of the above

121. True about internal anal sphincter is-
(A) middle part corresponds to pectinate line
(B) lower end corresponds to Hilton's line
(C) supplied by superior hypo gastric nerves
(D) all of the above

122. True about external anal sphincter is all except-
(A) voluntary sphincter
(B) surrounds upper $1/3^{rd}$ of anal canal
(C) surrounds whole of anal canal
(D) has three parts

123. Following are parts of external anal sphincter is all except-
(A) superficial part
(B) muco- cutaneous part
(C) subcutaneous part
(D) deep part

124. Part of external anal sphincter not attached to perineal body is-
(A) superficial part
(B) subcutaneous part
(C) deep part
(D) none of the above

125. External anal sphincter is supplied by-
(A) inferior rectal nerve
(B) perineal branch of 4th sacral nerve
(C) both a & b
(D) none

126. Part of external anal sphincter contributing to Anorectal ring is -
(A) superficial part
(B) subcutaneous part
(C) deep part
(D) all of the above

127. Anorectal ring is formed by-
(A) internal sphincter upper part
(B) internal sphincter middle part
(C) internal sphincter lower part
(D) all of the above

128. Anorectal ring is formed by-
(A) puborectalis muscle
(B) deep part of external anal sphincter
(C) upper part of internal anal sphincter
(D) all of the above

129. True about superficial part of external anal sphincter is-
(A) elliptical in shape
(B) arises from tip of coccyx & anococcygeal raphe
(C) inserted in perineal body
(D) all of the above

130. Incontinence of faeces occurs due to damage of-
(A) internal anal sphincter
(B) external anal sphincter
(C) anorectal ring
(D) all of the above

Answersheet

1. **D**	2. **D**	3. **C**	4. **D**	5. **A**	6. **D**	7. **C**	8. **D**	9. **D**	10. **D**
11. **C**	12. **C**	13. **D**	14. **B**	15. **A**	16. **B**	17. **C**	18. **D**	19. **C**	20. **B**
21. **B**	22. **D**	23. **C**	24. **A**	25. **D**	26. **E**	27. **B**	28. **E**	29. **D**	30. **B**
31. **D**	32. **D**	33. **D**	34. **D**	35. **B**	36. **C**	37. **B**	38. **B**	39. **C**	40. **B**
41. **B**	42. **C**	43. **D**	44. **D**	45. **D**	46. **C**	47. **D**	48. **B**	49. **C**	50. **D**
51. **D**	52. **D**	53. **D**	54. **A**	55. **D**	56. **D**	57. **B**	58. **D**	59. **C**	60. **B**
61. **C**	62. **A**	63. **B**	64. **C**	65. **B**	66. **C**	67. **B**	68. **A**	69. **B**	70. **C**
71. **C**	72. **D**	73. **C**	74. **D**	75. **C**	76. **C**	77. **C**	78. **D**	79. **B**	80. **A**
81. **C**	82. **B**	83. **B**	84. **C**	85. **D**	86. **D**	87. **C**	88. **D**	89. **A**	90. **A**
91. **C**	92. **B**	93. **A**	94. **D**	95. **A**	96. **C**	97. **B**	98. **C**	99. **A**	100. **A**
101. **C**	102. **D**	103. **D**	104. **A**	105. **B**	106. **C**	107. **B**	108. **B**	109. **D**	110. **D**
111. **C**	112. **B**	113. **B**	114. **C**	115. **C**	116. **D**	117. **D**	118. **C**	119. **C**	120. **D**
121. **D**	122. **B**	123. **B**	124. **A**	125. **C**	126. **C**	127. **A**	128. **D**	129. **D**	130. **C**

Chapter 4

Blood Vessels of Abdomen

1. Inferior vena cava in fetal life carries-
   (A) oxygenated blood
   (B) deoxygenated blood
   (C) mixed blood
   (D) all of the above

2. Inferior vena cava in adult life carries-
   (A) oxygenated blood
   (B) deoxygenated blood
   (C) mixed blood
   (D) all of the above

3. Inferior vena cava is formed in front of-
   (A) L2 vertebra
   (B) L3 vertebra
   (C) L4 vertebra
   (D) L5 vertebra

4. IVC opens into right atrium-
   (A) opposite to 5th costo-sternal joint right side
   (B) opposite to 6th costo-sternal joint right side
   (C) opposite to 7th costo-sternal joint right side
   (D) opposite to 8th costo-sternal joint right side

5. IVC pierces the diaphragm-
   (A) T 8 level through right crus of diaphragm
   (B) T 8 level through central tendon of diaphragm
   (C) T 10 level through right crus of diaphragm
   (D) T 12 level through central tendon of diaphragm

6. True about the valves in IVC is-
   (A) no valve at all
   (B) valve at formation of IVC
   (C) valve at the opening into right atrium
   (D) both c & d

7. IVC is crossed by all except-
   (A) 1st part of duodenum
   (B) 3rd part of duodenum
   (C) right gonadal vessel
   (D) left gonadal vessel

8. IVC is crossed by all except-
   (A) right common iliac artery
   (B) superior mesenteric vessels
   (C) inferior mesenteric vessel
   (D) right gonadal vessel

9. IVC is in posterior relation to-
(A) 1st part of duodenum
(B) head of pancreas
(C) 3rd part of duodenum
(D) all of the above

10. All are left relations of IVC except-
(A) abdominal aorta
(B) right crus of diaphragm
(C) left crus of diaphragm
(D) caudate lobe of liver

11. All are right relations of IVC except-
(A) second part of duodenum
(B) hepato-renal pouch of Morrison
(C) thoracic duct
(D) right ureter

12. Length of abdominal aorta is-
(A) 22cm
(B) 16cm
(C) 10cm
(D) 5cm

13. Abdominal aorta bifurcates at-
(A) T12
(B) L3
(C) L4
(D) L5

14. Abdominal aorta pierces diaphragm and enters abdominal cavity at-
(A) T8
(B) T10
(C) T12
(D) L1

15. Coeliac trunk arises at –
(A) T12
(B) L1
(C) L2
(D) L3

16. Smallest branch of coeliac artery is-
(A) left gastric artery
(B) common hepatic artery
(C) splenic artery
(D) none of the above

17. Largest branch of coeliac artery is-
(A) left gastric artery
(B) common hepatic artery
(C) splenic artery
(D) none of the above

18. All are branches from common hepatic artery except-
(A) right gastric artery
(B) left gastric artery
(C) gastro-duodenal artery
(D) posterior superior pancreatico-duodenal artery

19. Which of the following is called as artery of Wilkie's-
(A) supraduodenal branch of right gastric artery
(B) supraduodenal branch of gastroduodenal artery
(C) supraduodenal branch of superior pancreticoduodenal artery
(D) none of the above

20. Pancreatic branches from splenic artery supply all except-
(A) head of pancreas
(B) body of pancreas
(C) tail of pancreas
(D) all of the above

21. First branch of superior mesenteric artery is-
(A) superior pancretico-duodenal artery
(B) inferior pancretico-duodenal artery
(C) middle colic artery
(D) right colic artery

22. Superior mesenteric artery arises at –
(A) T12
(B) L1
(C) L2
(D) L3

23. Superior mesenteric artery crosses-
(A) 1st part of duodenum
(B) 2nd part of duodenum
(C) 3rd part of duodenum
(D) 4th part of duodenum

24. Superior mesenteric artery crosses-
(A) right psoas major
(B) right ureter
(C) inferior vena cava
(D) all of the above

25. True about the relations of splenic artery is all except-
(A) runs anterior to omental bursa behind the stomach
(B) runs posterior to omental bursa behind the stomach
(C) runs on upper border of body of pancreas
(D) runs on upper border of tail of pancreas

26. Splenic artery runs in-
(A) gastrosplenic ligament
(B) lieno-renal ligament
(C) omental bursa
(D) all of the above

27. Short gastric artery runs in-
(A) gastrosplenic ligament
(B) lieno-renal ligament
(C) omental bursa
(D) all of the above

28. All are branches of splenic artery except-
(A) pancreatic branches
(B) short gastric artery
(C) right gastro epiploic artery
(D) left gastro epiploic artery

29. Short gastric artery supplies-
(A) body of stomach
(B) fundus of stomach
(C) pyloric antrum of stomach
(D) gastro-duodenal junction

30. Structures crossed by left gastric artery are all except-
(A) left crus of diaphragm
(B) left psoas major muscle
(C) left sympathetic trunk
(D) left ureter

31. Structures crossed by left gastric artery are all except-
(A) left kidney
(B) left psoas major muscle
(C) left ureter
(D) left suprarenal gland

32. At origin of superior mesenteric artery splenic artery is-
(A) anterior to superior mesenteric artery
(B) posterior to superior mesenteric artery
(C) superior to superior mesenteric artery
(D) inferior to superior mesenteric artery

33. At origin of superior mesenteric artery left renal vein is-
(A) anterior to superior mesenteric artery
(B) posterior to superior mesenteric artery
(C) superior to superior mesenteric artery
(D) inferior to superior mesenteric artery

34. All are branches of superior mesenteric artery except-
(A) middle colic artery
(B) right colic artery
(C) ileo –colic artery
(D) left colic artery

35. Branches of ileo-colic artery are-
(A) anterior & posterior caecal artery
(B) appendicular artery
(C) ileal branch
(D) all of the above

36. Inferior mesenteric artery arises from abdominal aorta at-
(A) T12 Vertebra
(B) L1 Vertebra
(C) L2 Vertebra
(D) L3 Vertebra

37. At origin of inferior mesenteric artery–
(A) runs anterior to first part of duodenum
(B) runs posterior to first part of duodenum
(C) runs anterior to third part of duodenum
(D) runs posterior to third part of duodenum

38. Inferior mesenteric artery enters into lesser pelvis after crossing-
(A) left common iliac artery
(B) left internal iliac artery
(C) left external iliac artery
(D) none of the above

39. Branches of inferior mesenteric artery are-
(A) left colic artery
(B) sigmoidal arteries
(C) superior rectal artery
(D) all of the above

40. Continuation of superior mesenteric artery is-
(A) middle colic artery
(B) ileo-colic artery
(C) right colic artery
(D) left colic artery

41. Continuation of inferior mesenteric artery is-
(A) middle colic artery
(B) left colic artery
(C) right colic artery
(D) superior rectal artery

42. Left colic artery crosses-
(A) left psoas muscle
(B) left ureter
(C) left gonadal vessel
(D) all of the above

43. Marginal artery of Drummond extends from-
(A) superior to inferior mesenteric artery
(B) ileo caecal to left colic artery
(C) ileo caecal to recto sigmoid junction
(D) none of the above

44. Critical point of Sudeck is when-
(A) left colic artery fails to join middle colic artery
(B) lowest sigmoidal artery fails to join inferior rectal artery
(C) lowest sigmoidal artery fails to join superior rectal artery
(D) none of the above

45. When anastomosis between middle and left colic artery does not exist, there may be direct retroperitoneal anastomosis between trunks of superior and inferior mesenteric arteries called-

(A) Drummond's artery
(B) Sudeck's artery
(C) artery of Riolan
(D) none of the above

46. First paired arteries from abdominal aorta is-

(A) coeliac artery
(B) superior phrenic artery
(C) inferior phrenic artery
(D) renal artery

47. Right inferior phrenic artery crosses-

(A) inferior vena cava posteriorly
(B) inferior vena cava anteriorly
(C) anterior to esophagus
(D) posterior to esophagus

48. Left inferior phrenic artery crosses-

(A) inferior vena cava posteriorly
(B) inferior vena cava anteriorly
(C) anterior to esophagus
(D) posterior to esophagus

49. Inferior phrenic artery gives branch to supra renal gland as-

(A) superior supra renal artery
(B) middle supra renal artery
(C) inferior supra renal artery
(D) all of the above

50. Middle supra renal arteries arise at-

(A) T12 vertebral level
(B) L1 vertebral level
(C) L2 vertebral level
(D) L3 vertebral level

51. Middle supra renal arteries arise at the level of origin of-

(A) coeliac artery
(B) superior mesenteric artery
(C) inferior mesenteric artery
(D) none of the above

52. True statement about renal artery is-

(A) right renal artery is shorter than left
(B) right renal artery is longer than left
(C) right and left renal arteries are almost equal
(D) none of the above

53. True statement about renal artery is-

(A) right renal artery is higher than left
(B) right renal artery is lower than left
(C) right and left renal arteries are almost equal
(D) none of the above

54. Right renal artery is passes behind to–

(A) inferior vena cava
(B) head of pancreas
(C) second part of duodenum
(D) all of the above

55. Left renal artery is passes behind to all except –

(A) head of pancreas
(B) body of pancreas
(C) left renal vein
(D) splenic vein

56. Renal artery gives –

(A) superior supra renal artery
(B) middle supra renal artery
(C) inferior supra renal artery
(D) all of the above

57. Quadratus lumborum muscle is crossed by –
(A) 1st lumbar artery
(B) 2nd lumbar artery
(C) 3rd lumbar artery
(D) 4th lumbar artery

58. Quadratus lumborum muscle covers following arteries except –
(A) 1st lumbar artery
(B) 2nd lumbar artery
(C) 3rd lumbar artery
(D) 4th lumbar artery

59. Right gonadal artery is crossed by all except-
(A) third part of duodenum
(B) inferior vena cava
(C) root of mesentery
(D) ileum

60. Left gonadal artery is crossed by all except-
(A) left colic vessels
(B) root of mesentery
(C) inferior mesenteric vein
(D) descending colon

61. Common iliac arteries arise at-
(A) L2
(B) L3
(C) L4
(D) L5

62. True about common iliac arteries is-
(A) right & left common iliac arteries are equal
(B) right common iliac artery is shorter than left
(C) right common iliac artery is longer than left
(D) all are true

63. Posterior relations of right common iliac artery are-
(A) right psoas major muscle
(B) right & left common iliac veins
(C) formation of inferior vena cava
(D) all are true

64. Supra renal gland is supplied by -
(A) inferior phranic artery
(B) abdominal aorta
(C) supre renal artery
(D) all of the above

Answersheet

1. **C**	2. **B**	3. **D**	4. **B**	5. **B**	6. **C**	7. **D**	8. **C**	9. **D**	10. **C**
11. **C**	12. **C**	13. **C**	14. **C**	15. **A**	16. **A**	17. **C**	18. **B**	19. **B**	20. **A**
21. **B**	22. **B**	23. **C**	24. **D**	25. **A**	26. **B**	27. **A**	28. **C**	29. **B**	30. **D**
31. **C**	32. **C**	33. **D**	34. **D**	35. **D**	36. **D**	37. **D**	38. **A**	39. **D**	40. **B**
41. **D**	42. **D**	43. **C**	44. **C**	45. **C**	46. **C**	47. **A**	48. **D**	49. **A**	50. **B**
51. **B**	52. **B**	53. **B**	54. **D**	55. **A**	56. **C**	57. **D**	58. **D**	59. **B**	60. **B**
61. **C**	62. **C**	63. **C**	64. **D**						

Chapter 5

Nerves of Abdomen

1. Nervous furcalis is-
   (A) first lumbar nerve
   (B) second lumbar nerve
   (C) third lumbar nerve
   (D) fourth lumbar nerve

2. Lumbosacral trunk is formed by-
   (A) first & second lumbar nerve
   (B) second& third lumbar nerve
   (C) third & fourth lumbar nerve
   (D) fourth & fifth lumbar nerve

3. In prefixed lumbar plexus nervous furcalis is-
   (A) first lumbar nerve
   (B) second lumbar nerve
   (C) third lumbar nerve
   (D) fourth lumbar nerve

4. In postfixed lumbar plexus nervous furcalis is-
   (A) second lumbar nerve
   (B) third lumbar nerve
   (C) fourth lumbar nerve
   (D) fifth lumbar nerve

5. Root value of ilio-hypogastric nerve is-
   (A) L1
   (B) L2
   (C) L3
   (D) L4

6. Root value of ilio-inguinal nerve is-
   (A) L1
   (B) L2
   (C) L3
   (D) L4

7. Root value of genito-femoral nerve is-
   (A) L1-L2
   (B) L2-L3
   (C) L2
   (D) L4

8. Root value of lateral femoral cutaneous nerve is-
   (A) L1
   (B) L2
   (C) L1-L2
   (D) L2-L3

9. Umbilical area is supplied by-
   (A) T9 nerve
   (B) T10 nerve
   (C) T11 nerve
   (D) T12 nerve

10. Iliohypogastric nerve emerges out from-

(A) medial border of psoas major

(B) lateral border of psoas major muscle

(C) lateral border of quadratus lumborum muscle

(D) medial border of quadratus lumborum muscle

11. Iliohypogastric nerve pierces-

(A) internal oblique

(B) transversus abdominis

(C) external oblique

(D) none of the above

12. Iliohypogastric nerve runs between-

(A) internal oblique & external oblique

(B) transversus abdominis & internal oblique

(C) external oblique & transverse abdominis

(D) none of the above

13. Iliohypogastric nerve supplies-

(A) internal oblique, transverse abdominis& external oblique

(B) transversus abdominis & internal oblique

(C) external oblique & transverse abdominis

(D) none of the above

14. Transversus abdominis muscle is pierced by-

(A) Iliohypogastric nerve

(B) ilioinguinal nerve

(C) genito femoral nerve

(D) a & b both

15. Ilio inguinal nerve pierces-

(A) internal oblique

(B) transversus abdominis & internal oblique

(C) external oblique & transversus abdominis

(D) none of the above

16. Ilioinguinal nerve supply-

(A) internal oblique

(B) transversus abdominis & internal oblique

(C) external oblique & transversus abdominis

(D) none of the above

17. Genito-femoral nerve pierces-

(A) psoas major

(B) quadratus lumborum

(C) both

(D) none

18. True about genito-femoral nerve is-

(A) remains retroperitoneal

(B) pierces psoas major muscle

(C) nerve is crossed by ureter

(D) all of the above

19. Genital branch of genito-femoral nerve-enters inguinal canal through-

(A) through superficial inguinal ring

(B) through deep inguinal ring

(C) pierces through roof then enter

(D) none of the above

20. Genital branch of genitofemoral nerve supplies-

(A) cremaster muscle

(B) skin of scrotum

(C) skin of mons pubis and labium majus

(D) all of the above

21. Femoral branch of genitofemoral nerve –
(A) present in medial compartment of femoral sheath
(B) present in middle compartment of femoral sheath
(C) present in lateral compartment of femoral sheath
(D) none of the above

22. Root value of genitofemoral nerve is-
(A) L1
(B) L1L2
(C) L2L3
(D) L2

23. Root value of lateral femoral cutaneous nerve-
(A) L1L2
(B) L2L3
(C) L2
(D) L3

24. Largest branch of lumbar plexus is-
(A) sciatic nerve
(B) femoral nerve
(C) obturator nerve
(D) accessory obturator nerve

25. In abdomen femoral nerve supplies-
(A) iliacus
(B) pectineus
(C) both
(D) none

26. Femoral nerve in femoral sheath is a content of-
(A) medial compartment
(B) middle compartment
(C) lateral compartment
(D) none of the above

27. Femoral nerve is formed by-
(A) ventral rami of L2L3L4
(B) dorsal rami of L2L3L4
(C) ventral rami of L3L4
(D) ventral rami of L3L4L5

28. Obturator nerve is formed by-
(A) ventral rami of L2L3L4
(B) dorsal rami of L2L3L4
(C) ventral rami of L3L4
(D) ventral rami of L3L4L5

29. Accessory Obturator nerve is formed by-
(A) ventral rami of L2L3L4
(B) dorsal rami of L2L3L4
(C) ventral rami of L3L4
(D) ventral rami of L3L4L5

30. Accessory obturator nerve supplies-
(A) adductor magnus
(B) pectineus
(C) iliacus
(D) all of the above

31. Sympathetic trunks enter abdomen passing deep to-
(A) median arcuate ligament of diaphragm
(B) medial arcuate ligament of diaphragm
(C) lateral arcuate ligament of diaphragm
(D) crus of ligament of diaphragm

32. Sympathetic trunks enter pelvis passing deep to-
(A) external iliac artery
(B) internal iliac artery
(C) common iliac artery
(D) all of the above

33. Right sympathetic trunk lies-
(A) anterior to inferior vena cava
(B) anterior to abdominal aorta
(C) posterior to inferior vena cava
(D) not related to inferior vena cava

34. Left sympathetic trunk lies posterior to all except-
(A) pancreas
(B) 4th part of duodenum
(C) abdominal aorta
(D) inferior mesenteric artery

35. Lumbar sympathetic chain presents-
(A) two lumbar ganglia
(B) three lumbar ganglia
(C) four lumbar ganglia
(D) five lumbar ganglia

36. Lumbar sympathetic chain may have up to -
(A) three lumbar ganglia
(B) four lumbar ganglia
(C) six lumbar ganglia
(D) eight lumbar ganglia

37. Largest lumbar ganglion is
(A) 2nd lumbar ganglion
(B) 3rd lumbar ganglion
(C) 4th lumbar ganglion
(D) 8th lumbar ganglion

38. Preganglionic fibers for lower limbs are derived from-
(A) T6-T12 spinal segments
(B) T10-L2 spinal segments
(C) T10-L4 spinal segments
(D) L1-L4 spinal segments

39. Bilateral excision of lumbar part of sympathetic trunks may lead to-
(A) loss of erection
(B) loss of ejection
(C) loss of ejection & erection both
(D) none of the above

40. Lumbar sympathectomy is useful in-
(A) vasospastic disorders of pelvis
(B) vasospastic disorders of lower limbs
(C) musculoskeletal pains
(D) varicose veins

41. Lumbar splanchnic nerves usually are-
(A) three in number
(B) four in number
(C) five in number
(D) six in number

42. Coeliac plexus is joined by-
(A) first lumbar splanchnic nerve
(B) second lumbar splanchnic nerve
(C) first & second lumbar splanchnic nerves
(D) first to fourth lumbar splanchnic nerves

43. Intermesenteric plexus is joined by-
(A) first lumbar splanchnic nerve
(B) second lumbar splanchnic nerve
(C) first & second lumbar splanchnic nerves
(D) first to fourth lumbar splanchnic nerves

44. Superior hypo gastric plexus is joined by-
(A) first lumbar splanchnic nerve
(B) first & second lumbar splanchnic nerves
(C) second & third lumbar splanchnic nerves
(D) third & fourth lumbar splanchnic nerves

45. Solar plexus is another name of-
(A) brachial plexus
(B) coeliac plexus
(C) superior mesenteric plexus
(D) superior hypo gastric plexus

46. Coeliac plexus contains-
(A) pair of coeliac ganglion
(B) superior mesenteric ganglion
(C) aortico-renal ganglion
(D) all of the above

47. Right coeliac ganglion is-
(A) anterior to left crus of diaphragm
(B) posterior to inferior vena cava
(C) posterior to abdominal aorta
(D) posterior to splenic artery

48. Left coeliac ganglion is-
(A) anterior to left crus of diaphragm
(B) posterior to inferior vena cava
(C) posterior to abdominal aorta
(D) posterior to splenic artery

49. Greater splanchnic nerve have contribution from-
(A) T5-T9
(B) T10-T11
(C) T8-L1
(D) none of the above

50. Lesser splanchnic nerve have contribution from-
(A) T5-T9
(B) T10-T11
(C) T8-L1
(D) none of the above

51. Supra renal plexus have contribution from-
(A) T5-T9
(B) T10-T11
(C) T8-L1
(D) none of the above

Answersheet

1. **D**	2. **D**	3. **C**	4. **D**	5. **A**	6. **A**	7. **A**	8. **D**	9. **B**	10. **B**
11. **B**	12. **B**	13. **B**	14. **D**	15. **B**	16. **B**	17. **A**	18. **D**	19. **B**	20. **D**
21. **C**	22. **B**	23. **B**	24. **B**	25. **C**	26. **D**	27. **B**	28. **A**	29. **C**	30. **B**
31. **B**	32. **C**	33. **C**	34. **C**	35. **C**	36. **D**	37. **A**	38. **B**	39. **B**	40. **B**
41. **B**	42. **A**	43. **C**	44. **D**	45. **B**	46. **D**	47. **B**	48. **D**	49. **A**	50. **B**
51. **C**									

Chapter **6**

Male Genital System

1. Male reproductive gland is-
(A) testes
(B) prostate
(C) bulbourethral glands
(D) all of the above

2. True statement about testis is-
(A) right & left testis are at same level
(B) right testis is lower than left testis
(C) left testis is lower than right testis
(D) none of the above

3. Accessory sex glands are-
(A) testes & prostate
(B) prostate & bulbourethral glands
(C) testes & bulbourethral glands
(D) all of the above

4. Upper end of testis is-
(A) directed posteriorly
(B) directed laterally
(C) directed antero-laterally
(D) directed postero-laterally

5. Appendix of testes is a remnant of-
(A) Gartner's duct
(B) Mullerian duct
(C) Stenson's duct
(D) none of the above

6. Upper end of testis is overlapped by-
(A) head of epididymis
(B) body of epididymis
(C) tail of epididymis
(D) all of the above

7. Lower end of testis is overlapped by-
(A) head of epididymis
(B) body of epididymis
(C) tail of epididymis
(D) all of the above

8. Structures related to posterior border of testis are-
(A) body of epididymis
(B) vas deferens
(C) spermatic cord
(D) all of the above

9. Visceral layer of tunica vaginalis covers testis on all areas except-
(A) anterior border
(B) posterior border
(C) medial surface
(D) lateral surface

10. Sinus of testis is present on-
(A) anterior border
(B) medial surface
(C) lateral surface
(D) posterior border

11. Tunica albuginea covers the testis on-
(A) lateral surface
(B) medial surface
(C) posterior border
(D) all around

12. Mediastinum testis a part of –
(A) tunica vasculosa
(B) tunica vaginalis
(C) tunica albuginea
(D) all of the above

13. Mediastinum testis is located in testis in-
(A) anterior border
(B) posterior border
(C) medial surface
(D) lateral surface

14. Vascular membrane is-
(A) tunica albuginea
(B) tunica vaginalis
(C) tunica vasculosa
(D) all of the above

15. Canal of epididymis is lined by-
(A) flattened epithelium
(B) ciliated columnar epithelium
(C) pseudo stratified columnar ciliated epithelium
(D) all of the above

16. Efferent ductules is lined by-
(A) flattened epithelium
(B) ciliated columnar epithelium
(C) pseudo stratified columnar ciliated epithelium
(D) all of the above

17. Rete testis is lined by-
(A) flattened epithelium
(B) ciliated columnar epithelium
(C) pseudo stratified columnar ciliated epithelium
(D) all of the above

18. Arterial supply of testes comes from-
(A) testicular artery
(B) cremastric artery
(C) artery of the vas deferens
(D) all of the above

19. Arterial supply of testes comes from branches of -
(A) abdominal aorta
(B) vesical artery
(C) inferior epigastric artery
(D) all of the above

20. Pampiniform plexus of vein draining testes at superficial inguinal ring –
(A) 16-20 testicular veins
(B) 8-12 testicular veins
(C) 4 testicular veins
(D) 2 testicular veins

21. Pampiniform plexus of vein draining testes at deep inguinal ring –
(A) 16-20 testicular veins
(B) 8-12 testicular veins
(C) 4 testicular veins
(D) 2 testicular veins

22. Pampiniform plexus of vein draining testes at posterior abdominal wall-
(A) 8 testicular veins
(B) 4 testicular veins
(C) 2 testicular veins
(D) 1 testicular vein

23. Testicular vein drains into-
(A) renal vein
(B) inferior vena cava
(C) both A & B
(D) none of the above

24. Right testicular vein drains into-
(A) right renal vein
(B) inferior vena cava
(C) left renal vein
(D) right supra renal vein

25. Left testicular vein drains into-
(A) right renal vein
(B) inferior vena cava
(C) left renal vein
(D) right supra renal vein

26. Development of testis is apparent at-
(A) 5th week of intra uterine life
(B) 6th week of intra uterine life
(C) 7th week of intra uterine life
(D) 8th week of intra uterine life

27. Lymphatic drainage of testes is-
(A) superficial inguinal lymph nodes
(B) deep inguinal lymph nodes
(C) pre & para aortic lymph nodes
(D) all of the above

28. Nerve supply of testes is from-
(A) renal plexus
(B) aortic plexus
(C) T10 & T11 spinal segments
(D) all of the above

29. Canal of epididymis and vas deferens is derived from-
(A) mesonephric duct
(B) paramesonephric duct
(C) Mullerian duct
(D) all of the above

30. Rete cords and testes cords are canalised at the age of-
(A) 7th week of intra uterine life
(B) 7th month of intra uterine life
(C) 7th month of foetal life
(D) at puberty

31. Gubernaculum testes is proximally attached to-
(A) lower pole of testes
(B) peritoneum anterior to testes
(C) mesonephric duct
(D) all of the above

32. Gubernaculum testes is distally attached to-
(A) bottom of scrotum
(B) perineum & symphysis pubis
(C) anterior superior iliac spine &saphenous opening
(D) all of the above

33. Testes appears in iliac fossa at the age of-
(A) 4th week of intra uterine life
(B) 10th week of intra uterine life
(C) 4th month of intra uterine life
(D) none of the above

34. Testes appear at deep inguinal ring at-
(A) 6th month of intrauterine life
(B) 7th month of intrauterine life
(C) 8th month of intrauterine life
(D) 9th month of intrauterine life

35. Testes appear in inguinal canal at-
(A) 6th month of intrauterine life
(B) 7th month of intrauterine life
(C) 8th month of intrauterine life
(D) 9th month of intrauterine life

36. Testes appear in scrotal sac at -
(A) 6th month of intrauterine life
(B) 7th month of intrauterine life
(C) 8th month of intrauterine life
(D) the time of birth

37. Gubernaculum testis after birth forms–
(A) appendix of testes
(B) vaginal sac
(C) scrotal ligament
(D) tunica albuginea

38. Factors responsible for descent of testes are-
(A) gubernaculum testis
(B) intra-abdominal pressure
(C) intra-abdominal temperature
(D) all of the above

39. Factors responsible for descent of testes are-
(A) arched fibres of internal oblique
(B) uncurling of foetal curve
(C) foetal testosterone
(D) all of the above

40. Most important factor for descent of testes is-
(A) foetal testosterone
(B) gubernaculum testis
(C) intra-abdominal pressure
(D) all are important

41. Cryptorchism is a condition where testis is located in-
(A) retained in abdomen since birth
(B) in the perineum
(C) in femoral triangle
(D) all of the above

42. Length of vas deferens is-
(A) 12 inches
(B) 18 inches
(C) 25 inches
(D) 45 inches

43. Length of vas deferens is-
(A) 25cms
(B) 45 cms
(C) 15 cms
(D) 75 cms

44. Sperms are stored in-
(A) testis
(B) ampulla of vas deferens
(C) seminal vesicles
(D) all of the above

45. Arterial supply to vas deferens is artery to vas branch of-
(A) middle rectal artery
(B) inferior vesical artery
(C) testicular artery
(D) all of the above

46. Ampulla of vas deferens relation with seminal vesicle posterior to urinary bladder is-
(A) vas deferens is lateral to seminal vesicle
(B) vas deferens is medial to seminal vesicle
(C) vas deferens is posterior to seminal vesicle
(D) vas deferens is anterior to seminal vesicle

47. Seminal vesicle is supplied by-
(A) superior vesical & superior rectal artery
(B) inferior vesical & superior rectal artery
(C) inferior vesical & middle rectal artery
(D) superior vesical & middle rectal artery

48. Secretion from seminal vesicle contain-
(A) vesiculase enzyme
(B) fructose
(C) prostaglandin
(D) all of the above

49. Ejaculatory duct is-
(A) 2cms long
(B) 2 inch long
(C) 7.5 cms long
(D) none of the above

50. Secretions from seminal vesicle is-
(A) acidic in nature
(B) alkaline in nature
(C) neutral
(D) none of the above

51. Secretions from prostate is-
(A) acidic in nature
(B) alkaline in nature
(C) neutral
(D) none of the above

52. Metal specifically present in prostatic secretion is-
(A) copper
(B) zinc
(C) iron
(D) selenium

53. Prostatic secretion contains-
(A) acidic phosphatase
(B) fibrinolysin
(C) prostaglandin
(D) all of the above

54. False capsule of prostate –
(A) contains prostate & urinary bladder
(B) derived from visceral layer of pelvic fascia
(C) prostatic venous plexus lies deep to it
(D) all of the above

55. Prostatic venous plexus ,present in gap between true and false capsule
(A) present all around
(B) present anteriorly only
(C) present all around except posteriorly
(D) none of the above

56. Urethra passes through prostate in median plane-
(A) at junction of anterior& posterior 1/2
(B) at junction of anterior 1/3 & posterior2/3
(C) at junction of anterior 2/3 & posterior 1/3
(D) at junction of anterior ¾ & posterior ¼

57. Anatomically prostate has –
(A) 3 lobes
(B) 4 lobes
(C) 5 lobes
(D) none of the above

58. Surgically prostate has –
(A) 3 lobes
(B) 4 lobes
(C) 5 lobes
(D) none of the above

59. All are anatomical lobes of prostate are except-
(A) median lobe
(B) posterior lobe
(C) lateral lobe
(D) none

60. Surgical lobes of prostate are -
(A) anterior lobe
(B) posterior lobe
(C) lateral lobe
(D) all of the above

61. Median lobe of prostate is bounded by-
(A) ureter & seminal vesicles
(B) urethra & vas deferens
(C) urethra & ejaculatory ducts
(D) none of the above

62. Prostate contains –
(A) fibrous tissue
(B) glandular tissue
(C) muscular tissue
(D) all of the above

63. Outer zone of glandular tissue contains-
(A) main prostatic glands
(B) sub mucous glands
(C) mucous glands
(D) all of the above

64. Inner zone of glandular tissue contains-
(A) main prostatic glands
(B) sub mucous glands
(C) mucous glands
(D) all of the above

65. Intermediate zone of glandular tissue contains-
(A) main prostatic glands
(B) sub mucous glands
(C) mucous glands
(D) all of the above

66. Corpora amylacea is seen in-
(A) seminal vesicle
(B) prostate
(C) pancreas
(D) thymus

67. Prostatic glandular follicles are lined by-
(A) columnar epithelium
(B) pseudo stratified columnar epithelium
(C) columnar ciliated epithelium
(D) none of the above

68. Carcinoma of prostate affects mainly-
(A) outer glandular zone
(B) inner mucous zone
(C) both A & B
(D) none

69. Prostate is supplied by –
(A) inferior vesical artery
(B) middle rectal artery
(C) internal pudendal artery
(D) all of the above

70. Prostatic venous plexus receives blood from-
(A) prostate gland
(B) deep dorsal vein of penis
(C) vesical plexus
(D) all of the above

71. Blood from prostate is drained into-
(A) common iliac vein
(B) internal iliac vein
(C) external iliac vein
(D) all of the above

72. Prostate develops from-
(A) urogenital sinus
(B) genital ridge
(C) wolfian duct
(D) Mullerian duct

73. Bulbourethral glands are situated in –
(A) superficial perineal pouch
(B) deep perineal pouch
(C) both A & B
(D) none

74. Greater vestibular glands in females are situated in-
(A) deep perineal pouch
(B) superficial perineal pouch
(C) both A & B
(D) none

75. Bulbourethral glands open –
(A) membranous urethra
(B) prostatic urethra
(C) spongy urethra
(D) none of the above

76. Spermatic cord contains-
(A) vas deferens
(B) Pampiniform plexus of veins
(C) testicular artery
(D) all of the above

77. Spermatic cord is about –
(A) 5 cms long
(B) 7.5 cms long
(C) 5 inches long
(D) 7.5 inches long

78. Position of Vas deferens in spermatic cord in relation to other contents–
(A) anterior
(B) posterior
(C) superior
(D) inferior

79. Arteries present in the spermatic cord are-
(A) testicular artery
(B) artery of vas
(C) cremastric artery
(D) all of the above

80. Cremastric artery is a branch from-
(A) abdominal aorta
(B) inferior vesical artery
(C) inferior epigastric artery
(D) all of the above

81. Testicular artery is a branch from-
(A) abdominal aorta
(B) inferior vesical artery
(C) inferior epigastric artery
(D) all of the above

82. Artery to vas deferens is a branch from-
(A) abdominal aorta
(B) inferior vesical artery
(C) inferior epigastric artery
(D) all of the above

83. Scrotum develops from-
(A) genital ridge
(B) cloacal membrane
(C) genital swellings
(D) urogenital sinus

84. True statement about Dartos muscle is-
(A) subcutaneous muscle
(B) involuntary
(C) supplied by sympathetic nerves
(D) all of the above

85. External spermatic fascia is derived from-
(A) external oblique muscle
(B) internal oblique muscle
(C) transversus abdominis muscle
(D) none of the above

86. Internal spermatic fascia is derived from-
(A) external oblique muscle
(B) internal oblique muscle
(C) transversus abdominis muscle
(D) none of the above

87. Cremasteric fascia is derived from-
(A) external oblique muscle
(B) internal oblique muscle
(C) transversus abdominis muscle
(D) none of the above

88. Cremastric muscle is supplied by-
(A) ilio-inguinal nerve
(B) genital branch of genitofemoral nerve
(C) subcostal nerve
(D) ilio-hypogastric nerve

89. Cremastric muscle acts like –
(A) voluntary muscle
(B) involuntary muscle
(C) both
(D) none

90. Arterial supply of scrotum is-
(A) superficial external pudendal artery
(B) deep external pudendal artery
(C) posterior scrotal artery
(D) all of the above

91. Arterial supply of scrotum is from branches of -
(A) femoral artery
(B) internal pudendal artery
(C) both A & B
(D) none of the above

92. Cutaneous nerve supply of scrotal sac is from-
(A) ilio-inguinal & genitofemoral nerve
(B) pudendal nerve
(C) posterior femoral cutaneous nerve
(D) all of the above

93. Root of the penis is situated in-
(A) deep perineal pouch
(B) superficial perineal pouch
(C) both A & B
(D) none

94. Bulbospoingiosus muscle of penis is-
(A) unipinnate
(B) bipinnate
(C) multipinnate
(D) nonpinnate

95. Helicine arteries are seen in-
(A) vas deferens
(B) uterus
(C) penis
(D) cervix

96. Structures seen on dorsal surface of penis are all except-
(A) pair of deep dorsal vein of penis
(B) pair of dorsal arteries of penis
(C) pair of dorsal nerves of penis
(D) deep dorsal vein of penis

97. Tunica albuginea is seen –
(A) testis
(B) corpora cavernosa of penis
(C) corpora spongiosa of penis
(D) all of the above

98. Ligaments of penis are-
(A) fundiform ligament
(B) suspensory ligament
(C) both A & B
(D) none of the above

99. Ligament of penis attached to symphysis pubis is-
(A) suspensory ligament of penis
(B) fundiform ligament of penis
(C) both A & B
(D) none

100. Ligament of penis attached to linea alba is-
(A) suspensory ligament of penis
(B) fundiform ligament of penis
(C) both A & B
(D) none

101. Arterial supply of penis is by paired –
(A) artery of the bulb
(B) deep artery of penis
(C) dorsal artery of penis
(D) all of the above

102. Helicine arteries are branches from-
(A) artery of the bulb
(B) deep artery of penis
(C) dorsal artery of penis
(D) all of the above

103. Superficial dorsal vein of penis drains into-
(A) great saphenous vein
(B) great superficial vein bilaterally
(C) superficial external pudendal vein
(D) prostatic venous plexus

104. Deep dorsal vein of penis drains into-
(A) great saphenous vein
(B) great superficial vein bilaterally
(C) superficial external pudendal vein
(D) prostatic venous plexus

105. Penis develops from-
(A) genital ridge
(B) genital tubercle
(C) genital swelling
(D) all of the above

Answersheet

1. **A**	2. **C**	3. **B**	4. **C**	5. **B**	6. **A**	7. **C**	8. **D**	9. **B**	10. **C**
11. **D**	12. **C**	13. **B**	14. **C**	15. **C**	16. **B**	17. **A**	18. **D**	19. **D**	20. **C**
21. **D**	22. **D**	23. **C**	24. **B**	25. **C**	26. **C**	27. **C**	28. **D**	29. **A**	30. **B**
31. **D**	32. **D**	33. **C**	34. **B**	35. **C**	36. **D**	37. **C**	38. **D**	39. **D**	40. **A**
41. **A**	42. **B**	43. **B**	44. **B**	45. **B**	46. **B**	47. **C**	48. **D**	49. **A**	50. **B**
51. **A**	52. **B**	53. **D**	54. **D**	55. **C**	56. **B**	57. **A**	58. **C**	59. **B**	60. **D**
61. **C**	62. **D**	63. **A**	64. **C**	65. **B**	66. **B**	67. **A**	68. **A**	69. **D**	70. **D**
71. **B**	72. **A**	73. **B**	74. **B**	75. **C**	76. **D**	77. **B**	78. **B**	79. **D**	80. **C**
81. **A**	82. **B**	83. **C**	84. **D**	85. **A**	86. **C**	87. **B**	88. **B**	89. **B**	90. **D**
91. **C**	92. **D**	93. **B**	94. **B**	95. **C**	96. **A**	97. **D**	98. **C**	99. **A**	100. **B**
101. **D**	102. **B**	103. **B**	104. **D**	105. **B**					

Chapter **7**

Female Genital System

1. Ovary is-
(A) retro peritoneal
(B) intraperitoneal
(C) nonperitoneal
(D) none of the above

2. Ovary is covered by-
(A) squamous epithelium
(B) cubical epithelium
(C) columnar epithelium
(D) all of the above

3. In nulliparous female ovary is situated in-
(A) ovarian fossa above the pelvic brim
(B) ovarian fossa below the pelvic brim
(C) recto uterine pouch
(D) none of the above

4. In newborn female ovary is situated in-
(A) ovarian fossa above the pelvic brim
(B) ovarian fossa below the pelvic brim
(C) recto uterine pouch
(D) none of the above

5. Ectopic ovary may be seen in-
(A) femoral triangle
(B) inguinal canal
(C) labium major
(D) all of the above

6. Tubal end of ovary is related to-
(A) uterine tube
(B) ovarian fimbria
(C) suspensory ligament of ovary
(D) all of the above

7. Hilum of the ovary is present on-
(A) Anterior/mesovarian border
(B) posterior border
(C) tubal end
(D) uterine end

8. Line of Furre or white line of ovary is seen on-
(A) Anterior/mesovarian border
(B) posterior border
(C) tubal end
(D) uterine end

9. Bursa ovarica is seen at-
(A) anterior/mesovarian border
(B) posterior border
(C) tubal end
(D) uterine end

10. Posterior border of ovary is related to-
(A) uterine tube
(B) ureter
(C) internal iliac vessels
(D) all of the above

11. True about boundaries of ovarian fossa-
(A) obliterated umbilical artery- antero-superiorly
(B) external iliac vein - superiorly
(C) ureter & internal iliac vessels- posteriorly
(D) all of the above

12. Structures lying in floor of ovarian fossa –
(A) external iliac vessels
(B) internal iliac vessels
(C) obturator nerve & vessels
(D) ureter & uterine vessels

13. Blood supply of ovary is from-
(A) ovarian vessels
(B) uterine vessels
(C) both a & b
(D) none of the above

14. Ovarian artery is a branch of-
(A) uterine artery
(B) abdominal aorta
(C) internal iliac artery
(D) external iliac artery

15. Ovarian artery before supplying the ovary passes through-
(A) suspensory ligament of ovary
(B) mesosalpinx
(C) mesovarium of broad ligament
(D) all of the above

16. Ovarian vein drains into-
(A) inferior vena cava
(B) left renal vein
(C) both a & b
(D) none of the above

17. Right ovarian vein drains into-
(A) right renal vein
(B) right uterine vein
(C) inferior vena cava
(D) all of the above

18. Left ovarian vein drains into-
(A) left renal vein
(B) left uterine vein
(C) inferior vena cava
(D) all of the above

19. Sympathetic nerves supplying ovaries are-
(A) L10
(B) L10/L11
(C) L11
(D) L11/L12

20. Number of Primary ovarian follicles present in ovary in newborn-
(A) 1, 00,000
(B) 2, 00,000
(C) 40,000
(D) none of the above

21. Number of Primary ovarian follicles present in ovary at puberty-
(A) 1, 00,000
(B) 2, 00,000
(C) 40,000
(D) none of the above

22. Ovary develops from-
(A) medulla of genital ridge
(B) cortex of genital ridge
(C) both A & B
(D) none of the above

23. Ovary develops from genital ridge-
(A) cephalic part
(B) middle part
(C) caudal part
(D) all of the above

24. Suspensory ligament of Ovary develops from genital ridge-
(A) cephalic part
(B) middle part
(C) caudal part
(D) all of the above

25. Gubernaculum of Ovary is traversed by which part of genital ridge-
(A) cephalic part
(B) middle part
(C) caudal part
(D) all of the above

26. Uterine tube develops from-
(A) upper part of mesonephric duct
(B) upper part of paramesonephric duct
(C) mesonephric tubules
(D) all of the above

27. Uterus develops from-
(A) upper part of paramesonephric duct
(B) middle part of paramesonephric duct
(C) mesonephric tubules
(D) all of the above

28. Cervix and vagina develops from-
(A) upper part of para mesonephric duct
(B) lower part of paramesonephric duct
(C) middle part of paramesonephric
(D) all of the above

29. Duct of epoophoron is a remnant of -
(A) upper part of para mesonephric duct
(B) upper part of paramesonephric duct
(C) mesonephric duct
(D) all of the above

30. Tubules of epoophoron is a remnant of-
(A) upper part of mesonephric duct
(B) upper part of paramesonephric duct
(C) mesonephric tubules
(D) all of the above

31. Ligament of ovary develops from-
(A) gubernaculum of ovary
(B) gubernaculum of testes
(C) mesonephric duct
(D) paramesonephric duct

32. Round ligament of ovary develops from-
(A) gubernaculum of ovary
(B) gubernaculum of testes
(C) mesonephric duct
(D) paramesonephric duct

33. Length of Uterine tube is about-
(A) 10 inch
(B) 10 cms
(C) 12.5 inch
(D) 15 cms

34. Uterine tube is present in upper free margin of -
(A) medial ½ of broad ligament
(B) middle ½ of broad ligament
(C) medial ¾ of broad ligament
(D) medial ¼ of broad ligament

35. Uterine ostium of fallopian tube is –
(A) 1mm in diameter
(B) 1 cm in diameter
(C) 3 mm in diameter
(D) 3cm in diameter

36. Abdominal ostium of fallopian tube is–
(A) 1mm in diameter
(B) 1 cm in diameter
(C) 3 mm in diameter
(D) 3cm in diameter

37. Transport of ova to uterus from ovary via oviduct is facilitated by-
(A) Ciliary beats in oviduct
(B) peristalsis of oviduct
(C) longitudinal grooves in oviduct & fimbria
(D) all of the above

38. Intramural part of uterine tube is-
(A) 1mm in length
(B) 1cm in length
(C) 3mm in length
(D) 3 cm in length

39. Isthmus of uterine tube is-
(A) 1mm in length
(B) 1cm in length
(C) 3mm in length
(D) 3 cm in length

40. Ampulla of uterine tube is-
(A) 1 mm in length
(B) 1 cm in length
(C) 3 cm in length
(D) 5 cm in length

41. Infundibulum part of uterine tube is-
(A) 1mm in length
(B) 1 cm in length
(C) 3 cm in length
(D) 5 cm in length

42. Fertilization of ovum generally takes place in-
(A) infundibulum part of oviduct
(B) isthmus of oviduct
(C) ampulla of oviduct
(D) intramural part of oviduct

43. Widest part of fallopian tube is-
(A) infundibulum
(B) isthmus
(C) ampulla
(D) intramural part

44. narrowest part of fallopian tube is-
(A) infundibulum
(B) isthmus
(C) ampulla
(D) intramural part

45. Types of cells present in epithelium of oviduct/fallopian tube-
(A) ciliated columnar
(B) secretory cells
(C) intercalary cells
(D) all of the above

46. Arterial supply of uterine tube is through-
(A) uterine artery
(B) ovarian artery
(C) both A & B
(D) none of the above

47. Lymphatic drainage of uterine tube is-
(A) pre aortic group of lymph node
(B) lateral aortic group of lymph nodes
(C) superficial inguinal lymph nodes
(D) all of the above

48. Part of fallopian tube draining into superficial inguinal lymph nodes is-
(A) fimbriated end
(B) ampulla
(C) intramural part
(D) isthmus

49. Fallopian tube is supplied by sympathetic nerves derived from-
(A) T10 –T12 spinal segments
(B) T12 – L1 spinal segment
(C) L1 – L2 spinal segments
(D) T10 – L2 spinal segments

50. Fallopian tube is supplied by-
(A) pelvic splanchnic nerves
(B) vagus
(C) T10-L2 sympathetic nerves
(D) all of the above

51. Lateral part of fallopian tube is supplied by-
(A) pelvic splanchnic nerves & vagus
(B) vagus & T10-L2 sympathetic nerves
(C) T10-L2 sympathetic nerves, pelvic splanchnic nerves & vagus
(D) all of the above

52. Fallopian tube develops from-
(A) mesonephric duct
(B) paramesonephric duct
(C) both A & B
(D) none of the above

53. Fallopian tube develops from-
(A) Mullerian duct
(B) Gartner's duct
(C) Wolfian's duct
(D) none of the above

54. Length of uterus in nulliparous uterus is –
(A) 2.5 cms
(B) 5.0 cms
(C) 7.5 cms
(D) 10 cms

55. Length of cervix of uterus in nulliparous uterus is –
(A) 2.5 cms
(B) 5.0 cms
(C) 7.5 cms
(D) 10 cms

56. Length of body and fundus of uterus in nulliparous uterus is –
(A) 2.5 cms
(B) 5.0 cms
(C) 7.5 cms
(D) 10 cms

57. Body to cervix ratio of uterus in nulliparous adult female is-
(A) 3:1
(B) 2:1
(C) 1:2
(D) 1:3

58. Body to cervix ratio of uterus in childhood is-
(A) 3:1
(B) 2:1
(C) 1:2
(D) 1:3

59. Maximum width of uterus that is at fundus is-
(A) 2.5 cms
(B) 5.0 cms
(C) 7.5 cms
(D) 10 cms

60. Normal attitude of uterus is-
(A) ante version & ante flexion
(B) ante version & retro flexion
(C) retro version & ante flexion
(D) retro version & retro flexion

61. Angle of ante version is-
(A) 70°
(B) 90°
(C) 110°
(D) 140°

62. Ante version of uterus is an angle between-
(A) axis of uterus & axis of vagina
(B) axis of uterus & axis of cervix
(C) axis of cervix & axis of vagina
(D) none of the above

63. Ante flexion of uterus is an angle between-
(A) axis of uterus & axis of vagina
(B) axis of uterus & axis of cervix
(C) axis of cervix & axis of vagina
(D) none of the above

64. Angle of ante flexon is-
(A) 70°
(B) 90°
(C) 110°
(D) 125°

65. Long axis of uterus corresponds to-
(A) axis of pelvic inlet
(B) axis of pelvic outlet
(C) both A & B
(D) none of the above

66. Long axis of vagina corresponds to-
(A) axis of pelvic inlet
(B) axis of pelvic outlet
(C) both A & B
(D) none of the above

67. Ante version is maintained by-
(A) pull of round ligament
(B) pull of utero sacral ligament
(C) uterine musculature
(D) all of the above

68. Junction of mobile and immobile part of uterus is-
(A) cervix
(B) isthmus
(C) vagina
(D) none of the above

69. Uterine cavity is absent in-
(A) fundus of uterus
(B) body of uterus
(C) cervix of uterus
(D) none of the above

70. Lateral border of uterus is-
(A) peritoneal & related to uterine vessels
(B) nonperitoneal & related to uterine vessels
(C) peritoneal & not related to uterine vessels
(D) nonperitoneal & related to ovarian vessels

71. Lateral angle or cornua of uterus is related to-
(A) uterine tube
(B) uterine tube & ligament of ovary
(C) uterine tube & round ligament
(D) uterine tube, round ligament & ligament of ovary

72. Uterine cavity in reproductive life is lined by-
(A) simple columnar epithelium
(B) columnar ciliated epithelium
(C) pseudo stratified columnar epithelium
(D) pseudo stratified ciliated columnar epithelium

73. Uterine cavity in pre-puberty life is lined by-
(A) simple columnar epithelium
(B) columnar ciliated epithelium
(C) pseudo stratified columnar epithelium
(D) pseudo stratified ciliated columnar epithelium

74. Basal layer of endometrium is supplied by-
(A) straight arteries
(B) spiral arteries
(C) both A & B
(D) none of the above

75. Functional layer of endometrium is supplied by-
(A) straight arteries
(B) spiral arteries
(C) both A & B
(D) none of the above

76. Menstruation occurs due to-
(A) straight arteries
(B) spiral arteries
(C) both A & B
(D) none of the above

77. True about muscle arrangement in myometrium of uterus is -
(A) outer - longitudinal muscle layer
(B) middle – circular muscle layer
(C) inner – reticular arrangement
(D) all of the above

78. Stratum vasculare is name given to-
(A) outer - longitudinal muscle layer
(B) middle – circular muscle layer
(C) inner – reticular arrangement
(D) all of the above

79. Living ligature is the another name given to-
(A) outer - longitudinal muscle layer
(B) middle – circular muscle layer
(C) inner – reticular arrangement
(D) all of the above

80. Torus uterinus a transverse ridge is seen at-
(A) posterior surface of body of uterus
(B) posterior surface of body of cervix
(C) posterior surface on utero-cervical junction
(D) anterior surface of body of cervix

81. Isthmus a constriction is seen at-
(A) posterior surface of body of uterus
(B) posterior surface of body of cervix
(C) anterior surface on utero-cervical junction
(D) posterior surface on utero-cervical junction

82. Anterior surface of supra-vaginal portion of cervix is-
(A) peritoneal & related to urinary bladder
(B) non-peritoneal & related to urinary bladder
(C) peritoneal & related to ureter
(D) non peritoneal & related to urethra

83. Posterior surface of supra-vaginal portion of cervix is-
(A) peritoneal
(B) related to sigmoid colon & small intestine
(C) pouch of Douglas
(D) all of the above

84. Lateral margin of supra vaginal cervix is related to-
(A) Mackenrodt's ligament
(B) attachment of broad ligament
(C) ureter & uterine artery
(D) all of the above

85. External os of cervix in adults is-
(A) circular
(B) vertical
(C) transverse
(D) none of the above

86. External os of cervix in newborn is-
(A) circular
(B) vertical
(C) transverse
(D) none of the above

87. Number of vaginal fornicies around cervix are-
(A) two
(B) three
(C) four
(D) five

88. Non peritoneal fornix is-
(A) anterior
(B) posterior
(C) right lateral
(D) left lateral

89. deepest fornix of vagina is-
(A) anterior
(B) posterior
(C) right lateral
(D) left lateral

90. scrapings for hormonal study are taken from-
(A) anterior fornix
(B) posterior fornix
(C) lateral fornix
(D) from any where

91. cervical canal is lined by –
(A) simple columnar epithelium
(B) columnar ciliated epithelium
(C) stratified squamous epithelium
(D) all of the above

92. Ovula nebothi is seen in-
(A) ovary
(B) oviduct
(C) cervix
(D) vagina

93. Functional isthmus is formed by-
(A) upper 1/3rd of cervix
(B) middle 1/3rd of cervix
(C) lower 1/3rd of cervix
(D) none of the above

94. All ligaments are attached to cervix except-
(A) broad ligament
(B) Mackenrodt's ligament
(C) uterosacral ligaments
(D) pubocervical ligaments

95. Lower uterine segment is formed by-
(A) A upper 1/3rd of cervix
(B) middle 1/3rd of cervix
(C) lower 1/3rd of cervix
(D) none of the above

96. Prolapse of uterus may occur due to injury to-
(A) broad ligament
(B) Mackenrodt's ligament
(C) uterosacral ligaments
(D) pubocervical ligaments

97. Cardinal ligament is-
(A) broad ligament
(B) Mackenrodt's ligament
(C) uterosacral ligaments
(D) pubocervical ligaments

98. Fundus and body of uterus develops from-
(A) Mullerian duct
(B) mesonephric duct
(C) genital ridge
(D) all of the above

99. Lymphatics from body and fundus of uterus drain into-
(A) preaortic & lateral aortic lymph nodes
(B) external iliac lymph nodes
(C) superficial inguinal lymph nodes
(D) all of the above

100. Lymphatics from lateral angle of uterus drain into-
(A) preaortic & lateral aortic lymph nodes
(B) external iliac lymph nodes
(C) superficial inguinal lymph nodes
(D) all of the above

101. Lymphatics from cervix drain into-
(A) external iliac nodes
(B) internal iliac nodes
(C) sacral lymph nodes
(D) all of the above

102. Part of uterine tube not present in broad ligament is-
(A) ampulla
(B) intramural part
(C) isthmus
(D) fimbriated end

103. Anterior wall of vagina is-
(A) longer than posterior wall
(B) shorter than posterior wall
(C) equal to posterior wall
(D) none of the above

104. Anterior wall of vagina is related to-
(A) base of urinary bladder
(B) ureters terminal part
(C) urethra in lower part
(D) all of the above

105. Posterior wall of vagina is related to-
(A) recto-uterine pouch
(B) anal canal
(C) perineal body
(D) all of the above

106. Muscle acting as sphincter of vagina is-
(A) levator ani
(B) intrinsic muscles of vagina
(C) cardinal ligament
(D) all of the above

107. Type of epithelium seen in vagina is-
(A) transitional epithelium
(B) stratified squamous epithelium
(C) stratified squamous epithelium non keratinized
(D) stratified cuboidal epithelium

108. Vagina is supplied by-
(A) uterine artery
(B) internal pudendal artery
(C) middle rectal artery
(D) all of the above

109. Azygous vaginal artery is formed by branches of –
(A) uterine artery
(B) internal pudendal artery
(C) middle rectal artery
(D) all of the above

110. Lymphatic drainage from vagina is-
(A) internal iliac lymph nodes
(B) external iliac lymph nodes
(C) superficial inguinal
(D) all of the above

111. Nerve supply of vagina is from-
(A) sympathetic L1L2
(B) parasympathetic S2S3S4
(C) both A & B
(D) none of the above

112. Vagina develops from-
(A) urogenital sinus
(B) genital folds
(C) both A & B
(D) none of the above

113. Labia majora develop from-
(A) urogenital sinus
(B) genital folds
(C) genital swellings
(D) none of the above

114. Greater vestibular glands are situated in-
(A) vestibule of vagina
(B) superficial perineal pouch
(C) deep perineal pouch
(D) none of the above

Answersheet

1. **B**	2. **B**	3. **B**	4. **A**	5. **D**	6. **D**	7. **A**	8. **A**	9. **B**	10. **D**
11. **D**	12. **C**	13. **C**	14. **B**	15. **D**	16. **C**	17. **C**	18. **A**	19. **B**	20. **B**
21. **C**	22. **B**	23. **B**	24. **A**	25. **C**	26. **B**	27. **B**	28. **B**	29. **C**	30. **C**
31. **A**	32. **A**	33. **B**	34. **C**	35. **A**	36. **C**	37. **D**	38. **B**	39. **D**	40. **D**
41. **B**	42. **C**	43. **C**	44. **D**	45. **D**	46. **C**	47. **D**	48. **C**	49. **D**	50. **D**
51. **B**	52. **B**	53. **A**	54. **C**	55. **A**	56. **B**	57. **B**	58. **C**	59. **B**	60. **A**
61. **B**	62. **C**	63. **B**	64. **D**	65. **A**	66. **B**	67. **D**	68. **B**	69. **A**	70. **B**
71. **D**	72. **A**	73. **B**	74. **A**	75. **B**	76. **B**	77. **D**	78. **B**	79. **C**	80. **C**
81. **C**	82. **B**	83. **D**	84.	85. **C**	86. **A**	87. **C**	88. **A**	89. **B**	90. **C**
91. **D**	92. **C**	93. **A**	94. **A**	95. **A**	96. **B**	97. **B**	98. **A**	99. **D**	100. **C**
101. **D**	102. **B**	103. **B**	104. **D**	105. **D**	106. **A**	107. **C**	108. **D**	109. **D**	110. **D**
111. **C**	112. **C**	113. **C**	114. **B**						

Chapter 8

Urinary System - Kidney, Supra Renal, Ureter, Urinary bladder & Prostate

1. Supra renal glands are situated-
   (A) intraperiotenially
   (B) retroperitoneally
   (C) extraperitoneally
   (D) none of the above
2. Color of supra renal gland is-
   (A) brown
   (B) golden yellow
   (C) pinkish red
   (D) all of the above
3. False capsule of supra renal gland is formed by-
   (A) renal fascia
   (B) condensation of adrenal tissue
   (C) cortex of suprarenal gland
   (D) none of the above
4. True capsule of supra renal gland is formed by-
   (A) renal fascia
   (B) condensation of adrenal tissue
   (C) cortex of suprarenal gland
   (D) none of the above
5. Fetal suprarenal gland is about-
   (A) 1/2 of the kidney size
   (B) 1/3 of the kidney size
   (C) 1/30 of the kidney size
   (D) 1/20 of the kidney size
6. Adult suprarenal gland is about-
   (A) 1/2 of the kidney size
   (B) 1/3 of the kidney size
   (C) 1/30 of the kidney size
   (D) 1/20 of the kidney size
7. All are true about left supra renal gland except-
   (A) longer than right
   (B) higher than right
   (C) pyramidal in shape
   (D) semi-lunar in shape
8. Anterior surface of right suprarenal is related to all except-
   (A) inferior vena cava
   (B) superior duodenal flexure
   (C) bare area of liver
   (D) right crus of diaphragm

9. Right supra renal vein emerges from-
(A) apex of right suprarenal gland
(B) base of right supra renal gland
(C) medial border of right supra renal gland
(D) lateral border of right supra renal gland

10. Left t supra renal vein emerges from-
(A) apex of left suprarenal gland
(B) base of left supra renal gland
(C) medial border of left supra renal gland
(D) lateral border of left supra renal gland

11. Medial border of left supra renal gland is related to-
(A) left coeliac ganglion
(B) left inferior phrenic artery
(C) left gastric artery
(D) all of thc above

12. Medulla forms about-
(A) 1/2 of cortex
(B) 1/3 of cortex
(C) 1/10 of cortex
(D) 1/30 of cortex

13. Cortex of suprarenal gland surrounds the medulla at all places except-
(A) apex of the gland
(B) hilum of the gland
(C) apex & base of the gland
(D) apex, base & hilum of the gland

14. Thickest area of suprarenal cortex is-
(A) zona glomerulosa
(B) zona fasciculata
(C) zona reticulosa
(D) all are equal

15. Columnar cells are seen in which layer of suprarenal cortex-
(A) zona glomerulosa
(B) zona fasciculata
(C) zona reticulosa
(D) all are equal

16. Spongiocytes in suprarenal cortex are seen in-
(A) zona glomerulosa
(B) zona fasciculata
(C) zona reticulosa
(D) all of the above

17. Vitamin C rich area of suprarenal cortex is-
(A) zona glomerulosa
(B) zona reticulosa
(C) zona fasciculata
(D) none of the above

18. mineralocorticoids of suprarenal cortex are secreted from-
(A) zona glomerulosa
(B) zona fasciculata
(C) zona reticulosa
(D) b & c both

19. Superior supra renal artery is a branch of
(A) inferior phrenic artery
(B) abdominal aorta
(C) renal artery
(D) all of the above

20. Middle supra renal artery is a branch of
(A) inferior phrenic artery
(B) abdominal aorta
(C) renal artery
(D) all of the above

21. Inferior supra renal artery is a branch of
(A) inferior phrenic artery
(B) abdominal aorta
(C) renal artery
(D) all of the above

22. Supra renal gland is a supplied by
(A) inferior phrenic artery
(B) abdominal aorta
(C) renal artery
(D) all of the above

23. Right supra renal vein drains into-
(A) right renal vein
(B) inferior vena cava
(C) right gonadal vein
(D) all of above

24. Left supra renal vein drains into-
(A) left renal vein
(B) inferior vena cava
(C) left gonadal vein
(D) none of above

25. Accessory supra renal glands are seen in-
(A) broad ligament of uterus
(B) spermatic cord of testis
(C) mesenteries of gut
(D) all of the above

26. Kidney secret following hormones-
(A) 1-25-hydroxy cholecalciferol
(B) erythropoietin
(C) renin
(D) all of the above

27. Kidney are lying against –
(A) T12 – L3
(B) T12 – L2
(C) L1 – L3
(D) T12 – L4

28. True statement about kidneys –
(A) right kidney is lower than left kidney
(B) upper poles are closer than lower
(C) retroperitoneal organ
(D) all are true

29. Trans pyloric plane passes through-
(A) upper part of hilum of right kidney
(B) lower part of hilum of right kidney
(C) upper part of hilum of left kidney
(D) all of the above

30. Trans pyloric plane passes through-
(A) upper pole of right kidney
(B) lower part of hilum of right kidney
(C) upper part of hilum of left kidney
(D) lower part of hilum of left kidney

31. Fibrous capsule of the kidney is-
(A) condensation of fibrous stroma of kidney
(B) perinephric fat
(C) condensation of extra peritoneal tissue
(D) none of the above

32. Renal fascia of the kidney is-
(A) condensation of fibrous stroma of kidney
(B) perinephric fat
(C) condensation of extra peritoneal tissue
(D) none of the above

33. Space of Gerota of the kidney is occupied with-
(A) condensation of fibrous stroma of kidney
(B) perinephric fat
(C) condensation of extra peritoneal tissue
(D) paranephric fat

34. Fibrous capsule covers the kidney and lines-
(A) walls of renal sinuses
(B) sheath around minor & major calyces
(C) pelvis of ureter
(D) all of the above

35. True capsule of the kidney is-
(A) condensation of fibrous stroma of kidney
(B) perinephric fat
(C) condensation of extra peritoneal tissue
(D) paranephric fat

36. Renal fascia is continuous laterally with-
(A) transverse abdominalis muscle
(B) psoas fascia
(C) fascia transversalis
(D) peritoneum

37. Fascia of Toldt's is-
(A) anterior layer of renal fascia
(B) posterior layer of renal fascia
(C) fibrous capsule of kidney
(D) paranephric fat

38. Fascia of Zuckerkendl's is-
(A) anterior layer of renal fascia
(B) posterior layer of renal fascia
(C) fibrous capsule of kidney
(D) paranephric fat

39. Fascia of Gerota's is-
(A) condensation of fibrous stroma of kidney
(B) perinephric fat
(C) condensation of extra peritoneal tissue
(D) none of the above

40. Condensation of extra peritoneal tissue around kidney is called-
(A) renal fascia
(B) fascia of Gerota's
(C) false capsule of kidney
(D) all of the above

41. Suspensory ligament of supra renal glands is derived from-
(A) true capsule of kidney
(B) adipose capsule
(C) fascia of Gerota's
(D) fascia of Toldt's

42. Posterior relations of right kidney are-
(A) 11th rib
(B) 12th rib
(C) 11th & 12th ribs
(D) none of the above

43. Posterior relations of left kidney are-
(A) 11th rib
(B) 12th rib
(C) 11th & 12th ribs
(D) none of the above

44. Muscles present in posterior relation of kidney are-
(A) psoas major
(B) quadratus lumborum
(C) transverse abdominis
(D) all of the above

45. Posterior relation of kidney are –
(A) subcostal nerve & vessels
(B) ilio-hypogastric nerve
(C) ilio-inguinal nerve
(D) all of the above

46. Anterior relations of right kidney are all except-
(A) right supra renal gland
(B) 2nd part of duodenum
(C) 3rd part of duodenum
(D) hepatic area

47. All anterior relations of right kidney are non-peritoneal except-
(A) right supra renal gland
(B) 2nd part of duodenum
(C) jejunal area
(D) colic area

48. All anterior relations of right kidney are non-peritoneal except-
(A) right supra renal gland
(B) 2nd part of duodenum
(C) hepatic area
(D) colic area

49. Anterior relations of left kidney are -
(A) left supra renal gland
(B) gastric area
(C) splenic area
(D) all of the above

50. Anterior relations of left kidney are -
(A) left colic flexure & descending colon
(B) body of pancreas
(C) coils of jejunum
(D) all of the above

51. All anterior relations of left kidney are non-peritoneal except -
(A) left supra renal gland
(B) gastric area
(C) pancreatic area
(D) colic area

52. All anterior relations of left kidney are peritoneal except -
(A) splenic area
(B) pancreatic area
(C) jejunal area
(D) gastric area

53. Peritoneal area anterior to left kidney separated by lesser sac is-
(A) gastric area
(B) splenic area
(C) jejunal area
(D) gastric & splenic area

54. Peritoneal area anterior to left kidney separated by greater sac is-
(A) gastric area
(B) splenic area
(C) jejunal & splenic area
(D) gastric & splenic area

55. Left kidney is related to derivatives of-
(A) fore gut
(B) mid gut
(C) hind gut
(D) all of the above

56. Glands related to left kidney are-
(A) adrenal
(B) spleen
(C) pancreas
(D) all of the above

57. Right renal artery is-
(A) shorter than left renal artery
(B) longer than left renal artery
(C) almost equal to left renal artery
(D) no co-relation

58. True about renal vein is-
(A) left is longer than right
(B) left is shorter than right
(C) almost equal on each side
(D) none of the above

59. Left renal vein drains-
(A) left supra renal vein
(B) left gonadal vein
(C) left kidney
(D) all of the above

60. Sympathetic nerve supply to kidney is from-
(A) T6-T12
(B) T9-L1
(C) T10 –L1
(D) T12-L2

61. Permanent kidney is derived/ developed from-
(A) pronephros
(B) mesonephros
(C) metanephros
(D) all of the above

62. Pronephros develops in-
(A) cervical region
(B) cervical & thoracic region
(C) lumbo-sacral region
(D) thoraco-lumbar region

63. Mesonephros develops in-
(A) cervical region
(B) cervical & thoracic region
(C) lumbo-sacral region
(D) thoraco-lumbar region

64. Metanephros develops in-
(A) cervical region
(B) cervical & thoracic region
(C) lumbo-sacral region
(D) thoraco-lumbar region

65. Collecting part of kidney develops from-
(A) metanephric blastema
(B) uretric diverticulum
(C) both of above
(D) none of the above

66. Secretory part of kidney develops from-
(A) metanephric blastema
(B) uretric diverticulum
(C) both of above
(D) none of the above

67. During fetal life pelvic metanephric kidney is supplied by-
(A) median sacral artery
(B) common & internal iliac artery
(C) inferior supra renal artery
(D) all of the above

68. During fetal life iliac fossa metanephric kidney is supplied by-
(A) median sacral artery
(B) common & internal iliac artery
(C) inferior supra renal artery
(D) all of the above

69. During fetal life lumbar metanephric kidney is supplied by-
(A) median sacral artery
(B) common & internal iliac artery
(C) inferior supra renal artery
(D) all of the above

70. Derivatives of mesonephric duct in male are-
(A) efferent ductules of testis
(B) paradidymis
(C) ductus aberrant superior and inferior
(D) all of the above

71. Mesonephric duct in male forms -
(A) vas deferens
(B) canal of epididymis
(C) seminal vesicle & ejaculatory duct
(D) all of the above

72. Mesonephric duct in female forms -
(A) epoophoron
(B) tubules of paraphoron
(C) Gartner's duct
(D) all of the above

73. Commonest renal congenital abnormality is-
(A) pelvic kidney
(B) polycystic kidney
(C) floating kidney
(D) single kidney with double ureters

74. Length of ureter is-
(A) 2.5 inches
(B) 25 inches
(C) 25 cms
(D) 10 cms

75. Pelvis part of ureter is-
(A) formed within renal sinus
(B) formed by union of major calyces
(C) continues as abdominal part at lower pole of kidney
(D) all of the above

76. Capacity of pelvis of ureter is-
(A) 50 to 70 ml
(B) 15 to 25 ml
(C) 5 to 7 ml
(D) none of the above

77. Posterior relations of abdominal part of ureter are-
(A) tips of transverse processes of all lumbar vertebrae
(B) psoas major muscle
(C) genitofemoral nerve
(D) all of the above

78. All are anterior relations of right ureter except-
(A) right gonadal vessel
(B) 1st part of duodenum
(C) 2nd part of duodenum
(D) 3rd part of duodenum

79. All are anterior relations of right ureter except-
(A) right colic artery
(B) ilio colic artery
(C) root of mesentery
(D) all of the above

80. Anterior relations of right ureter are -
(A) 2nd part of duodenum
(B) 3rd part of duodenum
(C) terminal part of ileum
(D) all of the above

81. Anterior relations of left ureter are -
(A) left colic artery
(B) sigmoid mesocolon
(C) left gonadal vessels
(D) all of the above

82. Pelvic part of ureter in female forms-
(A) anterior boundary of ovarian fossa
(B) posterior boundary of ovarian fossa
(C) lateral boundary of ovarian fossa
(D) none of the above

83. First part or vertical part of ureter is posteriorly related to-
(A) sacro-iliac joint
(B) lumbosacral trunk
(C) internal iliac vessels
(D) all of the above

84. First part or vertical part of ureter is laterally related to all except-
(A) obturator nerve & vessels
(B) lumbosacral trunk
(C) inferior vesical artery
(D) middle rectal artery

85. Obliterated umbilical artery is-
(A) anterior to vertical part of ureter
(B) posterior to vertical part of ureter
(C) lateral to vertical part of ureter
(D) medial to vertical part of ureter

86. Pelvi-uretric junction corresponds with the-
(A) hilum of kidney
(B) lower pole of kidney
(C) pelvic brim
(D) entry of ureter in urinary bladder

87. Constrictions in ureter are-
(A) mechanical
(B) developmental
(C) both
(D) none

88. Muscle of Bell is derived from-
(A) outer longitudinal muscle of ureter
(B) middle circular muscle of ureter
(C) inner longitudinal muscle of ureter
(D) all of the above

89. Mucous membrane of ureter is thrown in-
(A) 4 vertical folds
(B) 5 vertical folds
(C) 6 vertical folds
(D) 7 vertical folds

90. Mucous membrane of ureter is-
(A) stratified squamous epithelium
(B) pseudo stratified cuboidal epithelium
(C) transitional epithelium
(D) stratified squamous epithelium keratinized

91. Lymphatic drainage of upper 1/3 of ureter is-
(A) para aortic lymph nodes
(B) common iliac group of lymph nodes
(C) internal & external iliac lymph nodes
(D) all of the above

92. Lymphatic drainage of middle 1/3 of ureter is-
(A) para aortic lymph nodes
(B) common iliac group of lymph nodes
(C) internal & external iliac lymph nodes
(D) all of the above

93. Lymphatic drainage of lower 1/3 of ureter is-
(A) para aortic lymph nodes
(B) common iliac group of lymph nodes
(C) internal & external iliac lymph nodes
(D) all of the above

94. In adults urinary bladder is –
(A) abdominal organ
(B) pelvic organ
(C) abdomino-pelvic organ
(D) none of the above

95. In children urinary bladder is –
(A) abdominal organ
(B) pelvic organ
(C) abdomino-pelvic organ
(D) none of the above

96. Nerve supply of ureter is-
(A) T12-L1
(B) S2-S4
(C) both a & b
(D) none

97. Muscle lying between posterior & middle layer of thoracolumbar fascia is-
(A) quadratus lumborum
(B) erector spinae
(C) internal oblique
(D) rectus abdominis

98. Muscle lying between anterior & middle layer of thoracolumbar fascia is-
(A) quadratus lumborum
(B) erector spinae
(C) internal oblique
(D) rectus abdominis

99. Thoraco lumbar fascia gives origin to-
(A) transversus abdominis
(B) internal oblique
(C) transversus abdominis & internal oblique
(D) internal oblique & external oblique

100. Lumbar plexus lies –
(A) posterior to psoas muscle
(B) anterior to psoas muscle
(C) within psoas muscle
(D) in psoas fascia

101. In children neck of urinary bladder lies at-
(A) upper border of pubic symphysis
(B) lower border of pubic symphysis
(C) ischeal spines of hip bones
(D) none of the above

102. In adults neck of urinary bladder lies at-
(A) upper border of pubic symphysis
(B) lower border of pubic symphysis
(C) ischeal spines of hip bones
(D) none of the above

103. Shape of Urinary bladder when empty resembles as –
(A) triangular
(B) tetrahedral
(C) ovoid
(D) all of the above

104. Shape of Urinary bladder when full resembles as –
(A) triangular
(B) tetrahedral
(C) ovoid
(D) all of the above

105. Capacity of urinary bladder in adults is-
(A) 120-320 ml
(B) 220-500 ml
(C) 320-800 ml
(D) none of the above

106. Mean capacity of urinary bladder in adults is-
(A) 120 ml
(B) 220 ml
(C) 320 ml
(D) 500 ml

107. Median umbilical ligament is attached to-
(A) neck of urinary bladder
(B) apex of urinary bladder
(C) base of urinary bladder
(D) prostate and urinary bladder

108. Median umbilical ligament is remnant of-
(A) intra-abdominal part of allantois
(B) remnant of urachus
(C) plexup of vesical veins
(D) condensation of pelvic fabcia

109. Posterior surface of urinary bladder in males is related to-
(A) recto vesical fascia & coils of intestine
(B) vas deferens
(C) seminal vesicles
(D) all of the above

110. Posterior surface of urinary bladder in females is related to all except-
(A) recto uterine pouch
(B) cervix of uterus
(C) vagina
(D) all of the above

111. Most fixed part of urinary bladder is-
(A) neck of urinary bladder
(B) apex of urinary bladder
(C) base of urinary bladder
(D) prostate and urinary bladder

112. In males neck of urinary bladder rests on-
(A) prostate
(B) urogenital diaphragm
(C) both a & b
(D) none

113. In females neck of urinary bladder rests on-
(A) prostate
(B) urogenital diaphragm
(C) both a & b
(D) none A lateral ligaments

114. True ligaments of urinary bladder are all except-
(A) lateral ligaments
(B) puboprostatic ligaments
(C) medial umbilical fold
(D) posterior ligaments

115. False ligaments of urinary bladder are all except-
(A) lateral ligaments
(B) median umbilical ligament
(C) medial umbilical fold
(D) median umbilical fold

116. Vesical venous plexus is seen in-
(A) lateral ligaments
(B) puboprostatic ligaments
(C) medial umbilical fold
(D) posterior ligaments

117. Neck of urinary bladder is fixed by-
(A) lateral ligaments
(B) puboprostatic ligaments
(C) medial umbilical fold
(D) posterior ligaments

118. Floor of retro pubic space is formed by-
(A) medial puboprostatic ligament
(B) lateral puboprostatic ligament
(C) median umbilical ligament
(D) lateral ligaments

119. Medial umbilical fold is covering over-
(A) obliterated umbilical artery
(B) urachus
(C) obliterated umbilical vein
(D) none of the above

120. Median umbilical fold is covering over-
(A) obliterated umbilical artery
(B) urachus
(C) obliterated umbilical vein
(D) none of the above

121. Uvula vesicae is small elevation produced by-
(A) median lobe of prostate
(B) lateral lobe of prostate
(C) medial lobe of prostate
(D) all of the above

122. Bar of Mercier seen in urinary bladder is-
(A) uretero-urethral ridges-
(B) inter uretric ridge
(C) both a & b
(D) none

123. Muscle of Bell seen in urinary bladder is-
(A) uretero-urethral ridges-
(B) inter uretric ridge
(C) both a & b
(D) none

124. True about trigone of urinary bladder is all expect-
(A) most fixed part of urinary bladder
(B) most dependent part of urinary bladder
(C) develops from endoderm
(D) develops from mesoderm

125. Arteries supplying urinary bladder are-
(A) superior & inferior vesical arteries
(B) obturator artery
(C) superior gluteal artery
(D) inferior gluteal artery

126. True about Vesical plexus of veins is-
(A) passes through posterior ligament
(B) drains into internal iliac veins
(C) communicates with prostatic venous plexus
(D) all of the above

127. True about root value of Nervi erigentes are-
(A) T11 –L2
(B) S2 S3 S4 somatic nerve
(C) S2S3S4 parasympathetic nerve
(D) none of the above

128. True about Nervi erigentes is-
(A) spinal micturition center
(B) motor to detrusor
(C) S2S3S4 parasympathetic nerve
(D) all of the above

129. Nerve motor to external urethral sphincter is-
(A) nervi erigentes
(B) pudendal nerve
(C) T11,T12,L1,L2. spinal sympathetic
(D) all of the above

130. True about sympathetic fibers of T11 – L2 is-
(A) inhibitory to detrusor & motor to sphincter vesicae
(B) inhibitory to detrusor & inhibitory to sphincter vesicae
(C) motor to detrusor & inhibitory to sphincter vesicae
(D) none of the above

131. Apex of urinary bladder develops from-
(A) lower ends of mesonephric ducts
(B) vesico-urethral part of cloaca
(C) proximal part of allantois
(D) distal part of allantois

132. In female Urethra is a passage for-
(A) urine only
(B) seminal fluid
(C) both a & b
(D) none

133. In male Urethra is a passage for-
(A) urine only
(B) seminal fluid
(C) both a & b
(D) none

134. Length of male urethra is-
(A) 25 cms
(B) 18-20 cms
(C) 15 cms
(D) 15 inches

135. Length of prostatic part of male urethra is-
(A) 3 cms
(B) 15 cms
(C) 18-20 cms
(D) 15 inches

136. Length of spongy part of male urethra is-
(A) 3 cms
(B) 15 cms
(C) 18-20 cms
(D) 15 inches

137. Length of female urethra is-
(A) 3 cms
(B) 4 cms
(C) 15 cms
(D) 18-20 cms

138. Length of membranous part of male urethra is-
(A) 3 cms
(B) 2 cms
(C) 4 cms
(D) 18-20 cms

139. Minimum breadth of male urethra is at –
(A) prostatic part
(B) membranous part
(C) spongy part
(D) external orifice

140. Maximum breadth of male urethra is at –
(A) prostatic part
(B) membranous part
(C) spongy part
(D) external orifice

141. Average breadth of male urethra is-
(A) 2mm
(B) 4mm
(C) 6mm
(D) 8mm

142. Most wide and dilatable part of male urethra is-
(A) prostatic part
(B) membranous part
(C) spongy part
(D) external orifice

143. Posterior wall or floor of prostatic urethra exhibits-
(A) prostatic sinuses
(B) urethral crest
(C) colliculus seminalis
(D) all of the above

144. Urethral crest is formed by-
(A) insertion of urethral muscles
(B) insertion of ureteral muscles of trigone
(C) opening of ejaculatory ducts
(D) none of the above

145. Colliculus seminalis or Verumontanum presents openings of –
(A) prostatic utricle
(B) ejaculatory ducts
(C) prostatic utricle, ejaculatory ducts & vas deferens
(D) prostatic utricle, ejaculatory ducts & prostatic glands

146. Male analogue of vagina is-
(A) prostate
(B) prostate utricle
(C) seminal vesicle
(D) all of the above

147. True about relations of membranous urethra is-
(A) surrounded by sphincter urethrae
(B) bulbourethral glands & their ducts on either side
(C) deep dorsal vein of penis anteriorly
(D) all of the above

148. Diameter of bulbar /spongy urethra is-
(A) 8mm
(B) 6mm
(C) 4mm
(D) 2mm

149. Ducts of bulbourethral glands open into-
(A) navicular fossa of bulbar urethra
(B) intra bulbar fossa of bulbar urethra
(C) not fixed but open anywhere in bulbar urethra
(D) all of the above

150. Littre's gland open in –
(A) navicular fossa of bulbar urethra
(B) intra bulbar fossa of bulbar urethra
(C) spongy urethra except navicular fossa
(D) all of the above

151. Valve of Guerin are seen in-
(A) prostatic urethra
(B) membranous urethra
(C) lacuna magna in spongy urethra
(D) none of the above

152. Male urethra is lined by-
(A) transitional epithelium
(B) stratified squamous epithelium
(C) stratified columnar epithelium
(D) all of the above

153. Male urethra up to colliculus is lined by-
(A) transitional epithelium
(B) stratified squamous epithelium
(C) stratified columnar epithelium
(D) all of the above

154. Male urethra spongy part up to terminal fossa is lined by-
(A) transitional epithelium
(B) stratified squamous epithelium
(C) stratified columnar epithelium
(D) all of the above

155. Terminal fossa of male urethra is lined by-
(A) transitional epithelium
(B) stratified squamous epithelium
(C) stratified columnar epithelium
(D) all of the above

156. External urethral orifice of male urethra is lined by-
(A) transitional epithelium
(B) stratified squamous epithelium
(C) stratified columnar epithelium
(D) all of the above

157. Arterial supply of urethra is from-
(A) inferior vesical artery
(B) middle rectal artery
(C) internal pudendal artery
(D) all of the above

158. Arterial supply of urethra is from-
(A) superior rectal artery
(B) middle rectal artery
(C) inferior rectal artery
(D) all of the above

159. Nerve supply of urethra is-
(A) L1 L2 sympathetic fibers
(B) S2S3S4 parasympathetic fibers
(C) pudendal nerve
(D) all of the above

160. True about female urethra is-
(A) 4cms long
(B) 6mm in width
(C) embedded in anterior wall of vagina
(D) all of the above

161. Female urethra is lined with-
(A) transitional epithelium
(B) stratified squamous epithelium
(C) stratified columnar epithelium
(D) all of the above

162. Female urethra is lined with-
(A) transitional epithelium
(B) stratified squamous epithelium
(C) stratified columnar epithelium
(D) both a & b

163. Narrowest and least dilatable part of male urethra is-
(A) prostatic part
(B) membranous part
(C) spongy part
(D) none of the above

164. Star shaped outline of urethral lumen is noted in-
(A) prostatic part
(B) membranous part
(C) spongy part
(D) none of the above

165. Fusiform outline of urethral lumen is noted in-
(A) prostatic part
(B) membranous part
(C) spongy part
(D) none of the above

166. Trapezoid outline of urethral lumen is noted in-
(A) prostatic part
(B) membranous part
(C) spongy part
(D) none of the above

167. True about internal urethral sphincter is-
(A) derived from bladder musculature
(B) innervated by sympathetic T11-L2
(C) involuntary in control
(D) all of the above

168. True about external urethral sphincter is-
(A) derived from sphincter urethrae
(B) innervated by pudendal nerve
(C) voluntary in control
(D) all of the above

169. Para urethral glands are homologous to-
(A) penis
(B) testis
(C) prostate
(D) all of the above

170. External urethral sphincter is-
(A) surrounds membranous part of urethra
(B) made up of sphincter urethrae
(C) supplied by S2S3S4
(D) all of the above

Answersheet

1.**B**	2. **B**	3. **A**	4. **B**	5. **B**	6. **C**	7. **C**	8. **D**	9. **A**	10. **B**
11. **D**	12. **C**	13. **B**	14. **B**	15. **A**	16. **B**	17. **C**	18. **A**	19. **A**	20. **B**
21. **C**	22. **D**	23. **B**	24. **A**	25. **D**	26. **D**	27. **A**	28. **D**	29. **A**	30. **D**
31. **A**	32. **C**	33. **B**	34. **D**	35. **A**	36. **C**	37. **A**	38. **B**	39. **C**	40. **D**
41. **C**	42. **C**	43. **A**	44. **D**	45. **D**	46. **C**	47. **C**	48. **C**	49. **D**	50. **D**
51. **B**	52. **B**	53. **A**	54. **C**	55. **D**	56. **D**	57. **B**	58. **A**	59. **D**	60. **C**
61. **C**	62. **B**	63. **D**	64. **C**	65. **A**	66. **B**	67. **A**	68. **B**	69. **C**	70. **D**
71. **D**	72. **D**	73. **B**	74. **C**	75. **D**	76. **C**	77. **D**	78. **B**	79. **D**	80. **D**
81. **D**	82. **B**	83. **D**	84. **B**	85. **C**	86. **B**	87. **B**	88. **C**	89. **C**	90. **C**
91. **A**	92. **B**	93. **C**	94. **B**	95. **C**	96. **C**	97. **B**	98. **A**	99. **C**	100. **C**
101. **A**	102. **B**	103. **B**	104. **C**	105. **A**	106. **B**	107. **B**	108. **B**	109. **D**	110. **D**

111. **A**	112. **A**	113. **B**	114. **C**	115. **A**	116. **D**	117. **B**	118. **A**	119. **A**	120. **B**
121. **A**	122. **B**	123. **A**	124. **C**	125. **C**	126. **A**	127. **C**	128. **D**	129. **B**	130. **A**
131. **C**	132. **A**	133. **C**	134. **B**	135. **A**	136. **B**	137. **B**	138. **B**	139. **D**	140. **A**
141. **C**	142. **A**	143. **D**	144. **B**	145. **D**	146. **B**	147. **D**	148. **B**	149. **B**	150. **C**
151. **C**	152. **D**	153. **C**	154. **A**	155. **B**	156. **B**	157. **D**	158. **B**	159. **D**	160. **D**
161. **B**	162. **D**	163. **B**	164. **B**	165. **A**	166. **C**	167. **D**	168. **D**	169. **C**	170. **D**

Part - 2
Lower Limb

Chapter **9**

Osteology

1. Dorsal component of hip bone is-
   (A) ilium
   (B) ischium
   (C) pubis
   (D) all of the above
2. Ventral component of hip bone is-
   (A) ilium & ischium
   (B) ischium & pubis
   (C) pubis & ilium
   (D) all of the above
3. Supra cristal plane passes through-
   (A) lower border of L3
   (B) lower border of L4
   (C) lower border of L5
   (D) lower border of L5/S1
4. Anterior superior iliac spine gives attachment to-
   (A) sartorius & rectus femoris
   (B) rectus femoris & ilioinguinal ligament
   (C) inguinal ligament & sartorius
   (D) none of the above
5. Anterior inferior iliac spine gives attachment to-
   (A) sartorius & rectus femoris
   (B) rectus femoris & ilioinguinal ligament
   (C) iliofemoral ligament & rectus femoris straight head
   (D) iliofemoral ligament & rectus femoris reflected head
6. Posterior superior iliac spine corresponds to-
   (A) S1
   (B) S2
   (C) S3
   (D) none of the above
7. Caudal end of sub arachnoid space corresponds at-
   (A) a S1
   (B) S2
   (C) S3
   (D) none of the above
8. Iliac crest is crossed transversely by-
   (A) lateral cutaneous branch of subcostal nerve
   (B) lateral cutaneous branch of iliohypogastric nerve
   (C) lateral cutaneous branches of dorsal rami of upper three lumbar nerve
   (D) all of the above

9. Part of acetabular cavity made by ilium is-
(A) upper 2/5
(B) lower 2/5
(C) anterior 1/5
(D) none of the above

10. Part of acetabular cavity made by ischium is-
(A) upper 2/5
(B) lower 2/5
(C) anterior 1/5
(D) none of the above

11. Part of acetabular cavity made by pubis is-
(A) upper 2/5
(B) lower 2/5
(C) anterior 1/5
(D) none of the above

12. Gap between anterior superior iliac spine & anterior inferior iliac spine gives way to-
(A) femoral branch of genito-femoral nerve
(B) lateral femoral cutaneous nerve
(C) lateral cutaneous branch of subcostal nerve
(D) none of the above

13. Greater sciatic foramen transmits –
(A) piriformis muscle
(B) obturator internus
(C) quadratus femoris
(D) all of the above

14. Structures passing above the piriformis –
(A) superior gluteal nerve
(B) superior gluteal nerve & vessels
(C) superior & inferior gluteal nerve & vessels
(D) inferior gluteal nerve

15. Structures passing below the piriformis are all except –
(A) sciatic nerve
(B) superior gluteal nerve
(C) nerve to quadratus femoris
(D) inferior gluteal nerve

16. Structures passing below the piriformis –
(A) nerve to obturator internus
(B) posterior cutaneous nerve of thigh
(C) pudendal nerve
(D) all of the above

17. Structures passing through greater sciatic foramen & enter into lesser sciatic foramen-
(A) pudendal nerve
(B) internal pudendal vessels
(C) nerve to obturator internus
(D) all of the above

18. Pre-auricular sulcus more conspicuous in-
(A) male
(B) female
(C) parous female
(D) none of the above

19. Obturator foramen in hip bone of female is-
(A) oval & smaller
(B) oval & larger
(C) triangular & smaller
(D) triangular & larger

20. Obturator foramen in hip bone of male is-
(A) oval & smaller
(B) oval & larger
(C) triangular & smaller
(D) triangular & larger

21. Horse shoe shaped articular surface of acetabulum is called lunate surface is absent-
(A) anteriorly
(B) posteriorly
(C) inferiorly
(D) superiorly

22. Lesser sciatic notch is occupied by-
(A) tendon of obturator externus
(B) piriformis
(C) tendon of obturator internus
(D) all of the above

23. Ischeal spine gives attachment to-
(A) levator ani muscle
(B) sacrospinaous ligament
(C) both a & b
(D) none of the above

24. Dorsal surface of ischeal spine is crossed by-
(A) pudendal nerve
(B) nerve to obturator internus
(C) obturator nerve
(D) nerve to quadratus femoris

25. Dorsal surface of ischium is related to-
(A) piriformis
(B) sciatic nerve
(C) nerve to quadratus femoris
(D) all of the above

26. Medial margin of ischeal tuberosity gives attachment to-
(A) sacrotuberous ligament
(B) ischiofemoral ligament
(C) iliofemoral ligament
(D) sacrospinaous ligament

27. Lateral margin of ischeal tuberosity gives attachment to-
(A) sacrotuberous ligament
(B) ischiofemoral ligament
(C) iliofemoral ligament
(D) sacrospinaous ligament

28. Pubic tubercle gives attachment to-
(A) inguinal ligament
(B) cremester muscle
(C) in males crossed by spermatic cord
(D) all of the above

29. Iliac tuberosity provides attachment to-
(A) interosseous sacroiliac ligament
(B) dorsal sacroiliac ligament
(C) iliolumbar ligament
(D) all of the above

30. Preauricular sulcus gives attachment to-
(A) ventral sacroiliac ligament
(B) piriformis
(C) obturator internus
(D) all of the above

31. Hip bone ossifies from-
(A) 3 primary & 7 secondary centres
(B) 3 primary & 5 secondary centres
(C) 3 primary & 3 secondary centres
(D) 3 primary & 1 secondary centres

32. Primary center for ilium appears at-
(A) second month of intrauterine life
(B) fourth month of intrauterine life
(C) fifth month of intrauterine life
(D) seventh month of intrauterine life

33. Primary center for ischium appears at-
(A) second month of intrauterine life
(B) fourth month of intrauterine life
(C) fifth month of intrauterine life
(D) ninth month of intrauterine life

34. Primary center for pubis appears at-
(A) second month of intrauterine life
(B) fourth month of intrauterine life
(C) fifth month of intrauterine life
(D) eighth month of intrauterine life

35. At puberty hip bone is ossified except for-
(A) tri-radiate cartilage
(B) iliac crest
(C) ischeal tuberosity
(D) all of the above

36. Secondary center for acetabulum –
(A) single secondary center at puberty
(B) two secondary center at puberty
(C) three secondary center at puberty
(D) none of the above

37. Secondary center for iliac crest –
(A) single secondary center at puberty
(B) two secondary center at puberty
(C) three secondary center at puberty
(D) none of the above

38. Secondary center for ischeal tuberosity–
(A) single secondary center at puberty
(B) two secondary center at puberty
(C) three secondary center at puberty
(D) none of the above

39. Ischiopubic ramus is fused at-
(A) 5 years
(B) 8 years
(C) 12 years
(D) none of the above

40. Hip bone is completely ossified by the age of-
(A) 20-25 years
(B) 25-35 years
(C) 35-45 years
(D) none of the above

41. Greater sciatic notch is wider in females & angle is equal or more than-
(A) 50°
(B) 75°
(C) 90°
(D) 1150

42. Sub pubic angler wider in females and angle is equal or more than-
(A) 50 – 55°
(B) 80 – 85°
(C) 110 – 120°
(D) 130 – 145°

43. Ischiopubic ramus is everted in –
(A) females
(B) males
(C) both
(D) none

44. Chilotic line in case of females has-
(A) smaller pelvic part
(B) larger sacral part
(C) larger pelvic & smaller sacral part
(D) larger sacral & smaller pelvic part

45. Longest bone of the body is-
(A) tibia
(B) fibula
(C) femur
(D) all are equal

46. Strongest bone of the body is-
(A) tibia
(B) fibula
(C) femur
(D) all are equal

47. Length of the femur is-
(A) 15 inch
(B) 18 inch
(C) 20 inch
(D) 22 inch

48. Head of the femur forms-
(A) 1/3rd of sphere
(B) 2/3rd of sphere
(C) 3/4th of sphere
(D) none of the above

49. Head of the femur is directed-
(A) medially, upwards & backwards
(B) medially, upwards & forwards
(C) medially, downwards & backwards
(D) medially, downwards & forwards

50. Neck shaft angle of femur in adults is-
(A) 90 degree
(B) 125 degree
(C) 160 degree
(D) none of the above

51. Neck shaft angle of femur in children is-
(A) 90 degree
(B) 125 degree
(C) 160 degree
(D) none of the above

52. Neck of femur is an extension of-
(A) epiphysis
(B) diaphysis
(C) metaphysis
(D) all of the above

53. Neck shaft angle in females is-
(A) lesser than males
(B) greater than males
(C) almost the same
(D) all of the above

54. Angle of femoral torsion is-
(A) 15 degrees
(B) 25 degrees
(C) 45 degrees
(D) none of the above

55. Femoral condyle which transmits greater part of body weight to tibia is-
(A) medial condyle
(B) lateral condyle
(C) both equally transmit
(D) none of the above

56. Muscle that is inserted at the apex of greater trochanter is –
(A) piriformis
(B) obturator internus
(C) obturator externus
(D) gluteus medius

57. Muscle that is inserted at the trochanteric fossa of greater trochanter is –
(A) piriformis
(B) obturator internus
(C) obturator externus
(D) gluteus medius

58. Muscle that is inserted on the upper rough impression of greater trochanter is –
(A) piriformis
(B) obturator internus with two gemelli
(C) obturator externus
(D) gluteus medius

59. Muscle that is inserted on the lateral surface of greater trochanter is –
(A) piriformis
(B) obturator internus
(C) obturator externus
(D) gluteus medius

60. Muscle that is inserted on the anterior surface of greater trochanter is –
(A) gluteus medius
(B) obturator internus
(C) obturator externus
(D) gluteus minimus

61. Apex of lesser trochanter gives attachment to-
(A) iliacus
(B) psoas major
(C) piriformis
(D) gluteus medius

62. Base of lesser trochanter gives attachment to-
(A) iliacus
(B) psoas major
(C) piriformis
(D) gluteus medius

63. Popliteus muscle arises from –
(A) popliteal groove of lateral condyle
(B) popliteal groove of medial condyle
(C) intercondylar area of femur
(D) none of the above

64. Nutrient artery of femur is –
(A) branch of 1st perforator artery
(B) branch of 2nd perforator artery
(C) branch of 3rd perforator artery
(D) branch of 4th perforator artery

65. Femur ossifies from –
(A) 1primary & 2 secondary centers
(B) 1primary & 3 secondary centers
(C) 1primary & 4 secondary centers
(D) 1primary & 5 secondary centers

66. Primary center for shaft of femur appears at-
(A) sixth week of intra uterine life
(B) seventh week of intra uterine life
(C) eighth week of intra uterine life
(D) ninth week of intra uterine life

67. Neck of femur ossifies from-
(A) at the end of ninth month of intrauterine life
(B) during first six months of life
(C) fourth year of life
(D) primary center for shaft

68. Secondary center for lesser trochanter of femur appears at-
(A) at the end of ninth month of intrauterine life
(B) during first six months of life
(C) fourth year of life
(D) twelfth year of life

69. Secondary center for greater trochanter of femur appears at-
(A) at the end of ninth month of intrauterine life
(B) during first six months of life
(C) fourth year of life
(D) twelfth year of life

70. Secondary center for lower end of femur appears at-
(A) at the end of ninth month of intrauterine life
(B) during first six months of life
(C) fourth year of life
(D) twelfth year of life

71. Secondary center for head of femur appears at-
(A) at the end of ninth month of intrauterine life
(B) during first six months of life
(C) fourth year of life
(D) twelfth year of life

72. Head and shaft of femur are fused at the age of-
(A) 16 years
(B) 18 years
(C) 20 years
(D) 22 years

73. Lower end and shaft of femur are fused at the age of-
(A) 16 years
(B) 18 years
(C) 20 years
(D) 22 years

74. Growing end of the femur is-
(A) upper end
(B) lower end
(C) shaft
(D) none of the above

75. Lower epiphyseal line passes through-
(A) medial condyle
(B) adductor tubercle
(C) lateral condyle
(D) all of the above

76. Largest sesamoid bone of the body is-
(A) patella
(B) fabella
(C) pisiform
(D) none of the above

77. Patella develops in the tendon of –
(A) triceps
(B) quadriceps femoris
(C) hamstrings
(D) all of the above

78. Articular area of patella is-
(A) upper 3/4th of posterior surface
(B) upper 2/3rd of posterior surface
(C) lower 3/4th of posterior surface
(D) lower 2/3rd of posterior surface

79. Articular area of patella is divided by vertical ridge and –
(A) has larger medial area
(B) has larger lateral area
(C) has equal lateral & medial area
(D) none of the above

80. Most common dislocations of patella are-
(A) medially
(B) laterally
(C) superiorly
(D) inferiorly

81. Tibia is homologous to –
(A) radius of forearm
(B) ulna of forearm
(C) none of the above
(D) both a & b

82. True about medial condyle of tibia is-
(A) larger than medial condyle
(B) articular surface is oval
(C) long axis is anteroposterior
(D) all are true

83. True about lateral condyle of tibia is-
(A) larger than medial condyle
(B) articular surface is circular
(C) long axis is anteroposterior
(D) all are true

84. Soleal line is present on –
(A) medial surface of tibia
(B) lateral surface
(C) posterior surface
(D) all of the above

85. Groove on posterior surface of medial malleolus gives attachment to-
(A) semitendinosus
(B) semimembranosus
(C) biceps femoris
(D) popliteus

86. Groove on posterior surface of lateral malleolus lodges -
(A) semitendinosus
(B) semimembranosus
(C) biceps femoris
(D) popliteus

87. Largest nutrient artery in human body is –
(A) nutrient artery of femur
(B) nutrient artery of tibia
(C) nutrient artery of humerus
(D) nutrient artery of radius

88. Nutrient artery to tibia is a branch from-
(A) popliteal artery
(B) posterior tibial artery
(C) anterior tibial artery
(D) none of the above

89. Tibia ossifies from-
(A) I primary & 2 secondary centres
(B) I primary & 3 secondary centres
(C) I primary & 4 secondary centres
(D) I primary & 5 secondary centres

90. Secondary center for upper end of tibia appears-
(A) first year of life
(B) just before birth
(C) just after birth
(D) fifth year of life

91. Secondary center for lower end of tibia appears-
(A) first year of life
(B) just before birth
(C) just after birth
(D) fifth year of life

92. Secondary center for lower end of tibia forms medial malleolus by-
(A) first year of life
(B) just before birth
(C) just after birth
(D) seventh year of life

93. Tibia represents-
(A) pre axial bone of leg
(B) post axial bone of leg
(C) both pre & post axial bones of leg
(D) none of the above

94. Upper end of tibia on media surface gives attachment to all except-
(A) sartorius
(B) gracilis
(C) semitendinosus
(D) semimembranosus

95. Fibula is homologous with-
(A) radius of forearm
(B) ulna of forearm
(C) both a & b
(D) none of the above

96. Tibia is homologous with-
(A) radius of forearm
(B) ulna of forearm
(C) both a & b
(D) none of the above

97. Muscles attached to medial surface of fibula are-
(A) extensor digitorum longus
(B) extensor hallucis longus
(C) peroneus tertitus
(D) all of the above

98. Muscles attached to posterior surface of fibula are-
(A) soleus
(B) flexor hallucis longus
(C) tibialis posterior
(D) all of the above

99. Head of fibula gives attachment to-
(A) biceps femoris
(B) semimembranosus
(C) tibialis posterior
(D) all of the above

100. Groove on posterior surface of lateral malleolus lodges-
(A) peroneus longus
(B) peroneus brevis
(C) peroneus tertitus
(D) a & b only

101. Nutrient artery enters fibula from-
(A) medial surface
(B) lateral surface
(C) posterior surface
(D) none of the above

102. Nutrient artery to fibula is a branch from-
(A) fibular artery
(B) peroneal artery
(C) anterior tibial artery
(D) posterior tibial artery

103. Pressure epiphysis in fibula is-
(A) upper end
(B) lower end
(C) both
(D) none

104. Neck of fibula is related medially to-
(A) common peroneal nerve
(B) anterior tibial vessels
(C) both a & b
(D) none of the above

105. Neck of fibula is related laterally to-
(A) common peroneal nerve
(B) anterior tibial vessels
(C) both a & b
(D) none of the above

106. Styloid process of fibula is present at-
(A) lower end
(B) upper end
(C) interosseous border
(D) none of the above

107. Deep peroneal nerve pierces-
(A) anterior intermuscular septa
(B) anterior intermuscular septa
(C) anterior intermuscular septa
(D) none of the above

108. Traction epiphysis in fibula is-
(A) upper end
(B) lower end
(C) both the ends
(D) none

109. Fibula ossifies from –
(A) one primary & one secondary centres
(B) one primary & two secondary centres
(C) one primary & three secondary centres
(D) none of the above

110. True about secondary center for upper end of fibula is-
(A) appears at 1st year & fuses on 18th year
(B) appears at 4th year & fuses on 18th year
(C) appears at 2nd year & fuses on 16th year
(D) appears at 1st year & fuses on 16th year

111. True about secondary center for lower end of fibula is-
(A) appears at 1st year & fuses on 18th year
(B) appears at 4th year & fuses on 18th year
(C) appears at 2nd year & fuses on 16th year
(D) appears at 1st year & fuses on 16th year

112. Superior tibiofibular joint is-
(A) syndesmosis
(B) plane synovial
(C) saddle type joint
(D) none of the above

113. Tarsals of foot are present in proximal row are –
(A) talus
(B) talus & calcaneum
(C) talus ,calcaneum & navicular
(D) none of the above

114. Tarsals of foot are present in distal row are –
(A) cuneiform & cuboid
(B) cuneiform, cuboid & navicular
(C) talus, calcaneum & navicular
(D) none of the above

115. Largest tarsal bone is-
(A) talus
(B) calcaneum
(C) navicular
(D) cuboid

116. Second largest tarsal bone is-
(A) talus
(B) calcaneum
(C) navicular
(D) cuboid

117. True about talus is-
(A) comma shaped facet laterally & large triangular facet medially
(B) comma shaped facet medially & large triangular facet laterally
(C) comma shaped facet anteriorly & triangular facet posteriorly
(D) circular facet laterally & triangular facet medially

118. Posterior facet on inferior surface of talus articulates with-
(A) anterior facet of calcaneum
(B) spring ligament
(C) middle facet of calcaneum
(D) none of the above

119. Anterolateral facet on inferior surface of talus articulates with-
(A) anterior facet of calcaneum
(B) spring ligament
(C) posterior facet of calcaneum
(D) none of the above

120. Medial facet on inferior surface of talus articulates with-
(A) anterior facet of calcaneum
(B) spring ligament
(C) posterior facet of calcaneum
(D) none of the above

121. Largest facet on inferior surface of talus is-
(A) anterolateral facet
(B) medial facet
(C) posterior facet
(D) none of the above

122. Neck body angle in of talus in adults is-
(A) 130
(B) 140
(C) 150
(D) none of the above

123. Neck body angle of talus in new born & infants is-
(A) 130 - 140
(B) 140 -150
(C) 150 -160
(D) none of the above

124. Long axis of neck of talus is directed-
(A) downwards, medially & forwards
(B) downwards, laterally & forwards
(C) upwards, medially & forwards
(D) none of the above

125. Trochlear surface of talus –
(A) superior surface
(B) articulates with tibia
(C) forms ankle joint
(D) all are true

126. Os trigonum may be a separate bone attached to –
(A) anterior surface of talus
(B) posterior surface of talus
(C) lateral surface of talus
(D) inferior surface of talus

127. Talus ossifies from one ossification center-
(A) appears at 6 week of intrauterine life
(B) appears at 3 months of intrauterine life
(C) appears at 6 month of intra uterine life
(D) appears at 6 month of life after birth

128. Groove on posterior surface of talus lodges-
(A) tendon of tibialis posterior
(B) tendon of flexor hallucis longus
(C) tendon of peroneus longus
(D) tendon of flexor digitorum longus

129. Long axis of calcaneum is directed-
(A) forwards, laterally & downwards
(B) forwards, upwards & laterally
(C) forwards, downwards & medially
(D) none of the above

130. Smallest surface of calcaneum is-
(A) anterior
(B) posterior
(C) superior
(D) inferior

131. Peroneal tubercle of calcaneum is present on-
(A) anterior surface
(B) lateral surface
(C) posterior surface
(D) medial surface

132. True about peroneal tubercle is-
(A) tendon of peroneus brevis passes above it
(B) tendon of peroneus longus passes below it
(C) tendon of peroneus tertitus passes below it
(D) both a & b are true
(E) all are true

133. Tendon passing deep to sustentaculum tali is-
(A) tibialis posterior
(B) flexor hallucis longus
(C) flexor digitorum longus
(D) none of the above

134. Tendon related medially to sustentaculum tali is-
(A) tibialis posterior
(B) flexor hallucis longus
(C) flexor digitorum longus
(D) none of the above

135. Calcaneum is ossified from-
(A) 1 primary & 1 secondary center
(B) 1 primary & 2 secondary centres
(C) 1 primary & 3 secondary centers
(D) 1 primary center only

136. Primary center for calcaneum appears at-
(A) 6 weeks of intra uterine life
(B) 3 months of intra uterine life
(C) 6 months of intrauterine life
(D) 3 months postnatally

137. Secondary center for calcaneum appears at-
(A) 6 - 8 months of intra uterine life
(B) 6 - 8 months life
(C) 6 - 8 years of life
(D) none of the above

138. Secondary center of calcaneum fuses with rest of bone at -
(A) 9 years
(B) 12 years
(C) 14-16 years
(D) 18-20 years

139. Boat shaped tarsal bone is-
(A) scaphoid
(B) talus
(C) navicular
(D) medial cuneiform

140. Tuberosity of navicular bone is present on-
(A) dorsal surface
(B) medial surface
(C) anterior surface
(D) plantar surface

141. Navicular bone ossifies from one center that appears at-
(A) 6 weeks of intrauterine life
(B) third month of intra uterine life
(C) third month of life
(D) third year of life

142. Smallest cuneiform bone is-
(A) medial cuneiform
(B) lateral cuneiform
(C) intermediate cuneiform
(D) none of the above

143. Largest cuneiform bone is-
(A) medial cuneiform
(B) lateral cuneiform
(C) intermediate cuneiform
(D) none of the above

144. Kidney shaped facet is present on medial cuneiform on-
(A) dorsal surface
(B) medial surface
(C) distal surface
(D) proximal surface

145. Lateral cuneiform ossifies from one ossification center –
(A) first year
(B) second year
(C) third year
(D) none of the above

146. Medial cuneiform ossifies from one ossification center –
(A) first year
(B) second year
(C) third year
(D) none of the above

147. Intermediate cuneiform ossifies from one ossification center –
(A) first year
(B) second year
(C) third year
(D) none of the above

148. Cuboid is ossified by one center that appears –
(A) 8 week of intrauterine life
(B) 3 months of intrauterine life
(C) just before birth
(D) just after birth

149. Cuboid articulates with-
(A) 4th metatarsal
(B) 5th metatarsal
(C) calcaneum
(D) all of the above

150. Longest among the metatarsals is-
(A) 1st metatarsal
(B) 2nd metatarsal
(C) 3rd metatarsal
(D) 4th metatarsal

151. Shortest among the metatarsals is-
(A) 1st metatarsal
(B) 2nd metatarsal
(C) 3rd metatarsal
(D) 5th metatarsal

152. Styloid process is lateral projection from the base of-

(A) 1st metatarsal

(B) 2nd metatarsal

(C) 4th metatarsal

(D) 5th metatarsal

153. 1st metatarsal ossifies from-

(A) 1 primary & 1 secondary center-

(B) 1 primary center

(C) 1primary center & 2 secondary centers

(D) none of the above

154. Primary center of ossification for 1st metatarsal appears at-

(A) 6th week of intrauterine life

(B) 8th week of intrauterine life

(C) 10th week of intrauterine life

(D) 12th week of intrauterine life

Answersheet

1. **A**	2. **B**	3. **B**	4. **C**	5. **C**	6. **B**	7. **B**	8. **D**	9. **A**	10. **B**
11. **C**	12. **B**	13. **A**	14. **B**	15. **B**	16. **D**	17. **D**	18. **C**	19. **C**	20. **B**
21. **C**	22. **C**	23. **C**	24. **B**	25. **D**	26. **A**	27. **B**	28. **D**	29. **D**	30. **D**
31. **B**	32. **A**	33. **B**	34. **C**	35. **D**	36. **D**	37. **B**	38. **A**	39. **B**	40. **A**
41. **B**	42. **B**	43. **B**	44. **C**	45. **C**	46. **C**	47. **B**	48. **B**	49. **B**	50. **B**
51. **C**	52. **B**	53. **A**	54. **A**	55. **B**	56. **A**	57. **C**	58. **B**	59. **D**	60. **D**
61. **A**	62. **B**	63. **A**	64. **B**	65. **C**	66. **B**	67. **D**	68. **D**	69. **C**	70. **A**
71. **B**	72. **B**	73. **C**	74. **B**	75. **B**	76. **A**	77. **B**	78. **A**	79. **B**	80. **B**
81. **A**	82. **D**	83. **B**	84. **C**	85. **B**	86. **D**	87. **B**	88. **B**	89. **A**	90. **B**
91. **A**	92. **D**	93. **A**	94. **D**	95. **B**	96. **A**	97. **D**	98. **D**	99. **A**	100. **D**
101. **C**	102. **B**	103. **B**	104. **B**	105. **A**	106. **B**	107. **A**	108. **A**	109. **B**	110. **B**
111. **D**	112. **B**	113. **B**	114. **A**	115. **B**	116. **A**	117. **B**	118. **C**	119. **A**	120. **B**
121. **C**	122. **C**	123. **A**	124. **A**	125. **D**	126. **B**	127. **C**	128. **B**	129. **B**	130. **A**
131. **B**	132. **D**	133. **B**	134. **C**	135. **A**	136. **B**	137. **C**	138. **C**	139. **C**	140. **B**
141. **D**	142. **C**	143. **A**	144. **C**	145. **A**	146. **B**	147. **C**	148. **C**	149. **D**	150. **B**
151. **A**	152. **D**	153. **A**	154. **C**						

Chapter **10**

Gluteal Region

1. Posterior superior iliac spine lies at –
(A) S1 spine
(B) S2 spine
(C) S3 spine
(D) S4 spine

2. Deep fascia of gluteal region encloses-
(A) gluteus maximus muscle
(B) tensor fascia lata muscle
(C) both a & b
(D) none of the above

3. All are supplied by superior gluteal nerve except-
(A) gluteus minimus
(B) gluteus medius
(C) gluteus maximus
(D) tensor fascia lata

4. Highest point of iliac crest corresponds-
(A) 2nd lumbar spine
(B) 3rd lumbar spine
(C) 4th lumbar spine
(D) 5th lumbar spine

5. Skin of gluteal region is supplied by-
(A) T12 ,L1 dermatome
(B) L2 dermatome
(C) S1,S2 & S3 dermatome
(D) all of the above

6. Skin of gluteal region is supplied by all except-
(A) T12 ,L1 dermatome
(B) L2 dermatome
(C) L3 L4 dermatome
(D) S1,S2 & S3 dermatome

7. Bursa related to gluteus maximus are-
(A) trochanteric bursa
(B) gluteo-femoral bursa
(C) ischeal bursa
(D) all of the above

8. Action of paradox is noted in-
(A) gluteus minimus
(B) gluteus medius
(C) gluteus maximus
(D) all of the above

9. Action of gluteus maximus is-
(A) extensor of hip
(B) lateral rotator at hip
(C) abductor of hip
(D) all of the above

10. Ilio tibial tract gets insertion of-
(A) tensor fascia lata
(B) gluteus maximus
(C) both a & b
(D) none of the above

11. Nerve supply of gluteus maximus is-
(A) superior gluteal nerve
(B) inferior gluteal nerve
(C) both a & b
(D) none of the above

12. Tensor fascia lata is supplied by-
(A) superior gluteal nerve
(B) inferior gluteal nerve
(C) both a & b
(D) none of the above

13. Inferior gluteal nerve supplies-
(A) gluteus minimus
(B) gluteus medius
(C) gluteus maximus
(D) tensor fascia lata

14. Superior gluteal nerve supplies-
(A) gluteus minimus
(B) gluteus medius
(C) tensor fascia lata
(D) all of the above

15. Structures coming out from greater sciatic foramen below piriformis-
(A) sciatic nerve
(B) posterior cutaneous nerve of thigh
(C) inferior gluteal nerve and vessels
(D) all of the above

16. Structures coming out from greater sciatic foramen below piriformis & entering through lesser sciatic foramen-
(A) nerve to obturator internus
(B) internal pudendal vessels
(C) pudendal nerve
(D) all of the above

17. Superior gamellus is supplied by-
(A) nerve to obturator internus
(B) nerve to quadratus femoris
(C) both a & b
(D) none of the above

18. Inferior gamellus is supplied by-
(A) nerve to obturator internus
(B) nerve to quadratus femoris
(C) both a & b
(D) none of the above

19. Tricipital tendon comprises of all except-
(A) gamellus superior
(B) obturator internus
(C) obturator externus
(D) gamellus inferior

20. Root value of superior gluteal nerve-
(A) L4L5S1
(B) L5S1 S2
(C) L4L5 S1 S2
(D) L3L4 L5S1

21. Root value of inferior gluteal nerve-
(A) L4L5S1
(B) L5S1 S2
(C) L4L5 S1 S2
(D) L3L4 L5S1

22. Root value of sciatic nerve-
(A) L4L5S1
(B) L5S1 S2
(C) L4L5 S1 S2S3
(D) L3L4 L5S1

23. Root value of nerve to quadratus femoris-
(A) L4L5S1
(B) L5S1 S2
(C) L4L5 S1 S2S3
(D) L3L4 L5S1

24. Gluteus muscle which is not abductor is-
(A) gluteus maximus
(B) gluteus minimus
(C) gluteus medius
(D) none of the above

25. Artery to sciatic nerve is a branch from-
(A) internal iliac artery
(B) superior gluteal artery
(C) inferior gluteal artery
(D) all of the above

26. Arteries raking part in cruciate anastomosis are all except –
(A) superior gluteal artery
(B) inferior gluteal artery
(C) first perforator artery
(D) branches from circumflex femoral arteries

27. Arteries raking part in trochanteric anastomosis are all except –
(A) superior gluteal artery
(B) inferior gluteal artery
(C) branches from circumflex femoral arteries
(D) all of the above

28. Gluteal region communicates with-
(A) pelvic cavity
(B) ischiorectal fossa
(C) posterior compartment of thigh
(D) all of the above

29. Gluteal region communicates with pelvic cavity through-
(A) greater sciatic foramen
(B) lesser sciatic foramen
(C) obturator foramen
(D) all of the above

30. Gluteal region communicates with ischiorectal fossa through-
(A) greater sciatic foramen
(B) lesser sciatic foramen
(C) obturator foramen
(D) all of the above

31. Deep fascia of gluteal region splits and encloses-
(A) gluteus maximus
(B) glutcus medius
(C) gluteus minimus
(D) all of the above

32. Deep fascia of gluteal region splits and encloses –
(A) tensor fascia lata
(B) gluteus medius
(C) gluteus minimus
(D) all of the above

33. Sacrotuberous ligament is supposed to be a part of-
(A) semi membranous
(B) semitendinosus
(C) biceps femoris
(D) adductor magnus

34. Sacrospinous ligament is supposed to be a part of-
(A) obturator internus
(B) coccygeus
(C) levator ani
(D) obturator externus

35. Apex of sacrospinous ligament crossed by -
(A) superior gluteal nerve
(B) pudendal nerve
(C) sciatic nerve
(D) inferior gluteal nerve

36. Weaver's bottom is inflammation of-
(A) trochanteric bursa
(B) ischeal bursa
(C) gluteofemoral bursa
(D) all of the above

37. Trendelberg's test is done to check-
(A) gluteus minimus
(B) gluteus minimus & gluteus medius
(C) gluteus minimus, gluteus medius & gluteus maximus
(D) gluteus minimus, gluteus medius & tensor fascia late

38. Muscle present in gluteal region & pelvis both is-
(A) superior gamellus
(B) piriformis
(C) quadratus femoris
(D) obturator externus

39. Posterior cutaneous nerve of thigh supplies skin of-
(A) inferolateral part of gluteal region
(B) scrotal area
(C) back of thigh & popliteal fossa
(D) all of the above

40. In gluteal region intra muscular injections are safely given in-
(A) superomedial quadrant
(B) superolateral quadrant
(C) inferomedial quadrant
(D) inferolateral quadrant

Answersheet

1. **B**	2. **C**	3. **C**	4. **C**	5. **D**	6. **C**	7. **D**	8. **C**	9. **D**	10. **C**
11. **B**	12. **A**	13. **C**	14. **D**	15. **D**	16. **D**	17. **A**	18. **B**	19. **C**	20. **A**
21. **B**	22. **C**	23. **A**	24. **A**	25. **C**	26. **A**	27. **D**	28. **D**	29. **A**	30. **B**
31. **A**	32. **A**	33. **C**	34. **B**	35. **B**	36. **B**	37. **B**	38. **B**	39. **D**	40. **B**

Chapter **11**

Front of Thigh

1. Skin overlying the femoral triangle is supplied by-
   (A) ilio-inguinal nerve
   (B) femoral branch of genito-femoral nerve
   (C) genital branch of genito-femoral nerve
   (D) both a & b
   (E) all of the above

2. Nerve emerging through superficial inguinal ring is-
   (A) femoral branch of genito femoral nerve
   (B) ilioinguinal nerve
   (C) iliohypogastric nerve
   (D) all of the above

3. Nerve emerging after piercing through femoral sheath is-
   (A) femoral branch of genito femoral nerve
   (B) ilioinguinal nerve
   (C) iliohypogastric nerve
   (D) all of the above

4. Root value of lateral femoral cutaneous nerve is-
   (A) L1L2
   (B) L2L3
   (C) L3L4
   (D) L2L3L4

5. Root value of posterior branch of lateral femoral cutaneous nerve is-
   (A) L1
   (B) L2
   (C) L3L4
   (D) L2L3L4

6. Root value of anterior branch of lateral femoral cutaneous nerve is-
   (A) L2
   (B) L3
   (C) L3L4
   (D) L2L3L4

7. Meralgia parasthetica is due to involvement of-
   (A) femoral branch of genito femoral nerve
   (B) ilioinguinal nerve
   (C) iliohypogastric nerve
   (D) lateral femoral cutaneous nerve of thigh

8. Root value of genito femoral nerve is-
(A) L2L3
(B) L1L2
(C) L3L4
(D) L2L3L4

9. Genital branch of genitofemoral nerve conveys fibers from-
(A) L1
(B) L2
CL1 L2
(D) L2L3L4

10. Femoral branch of genitofemoral nerve conveys fibers from-
(A) L1
(B) L2
CL1 L2
(D) L2L3L4

11. Nerve piercing the psoas major muscle is-
(A) lateral femoral cutaneous nerve of thigh
(B) genitofemoral nerve
(C) ilioinguinal nerve
(D) all of the above

12. Genital branch of genitofemoral nerve supplies-
(A) cremester muscle
(B) skin of scrotum
(C) mons pubis & labium majus
(D) all of the above

13. True about ilioinguinal nerve is-
(A) collateral branch of iliohypogastric nerve
(B) root value is L1
(C) remains in inguinal canal
(D) all of the above

14. Ilioinguinal nerve supplies skin of -
(A) front of thigh
(B) root of penis
(C) upper part of scrotum/labium majus
(D) all of the above

15. Pre axial vein of lower limb is-
(A) femoral vein
(B) great saphenous vein
(C) small saphenous vein
(D) popliteal vein

16. Post axial vein of lower limb is-
(A) femoral vein
(B) great saphenous vein
(C) small saphenous vein
(D) popliteal vein

17. Longest vein of the body is-
(A) femoral vein
(B) great saphenous vein
(C) small saphenous vein
(D) popliteal vein

18. Great saphenous vein starts as-
(A) continuation as lateral end of dorsal venous arch of foot
(B) continuation of medial end of dorsal venous arch of foot
(C) supplemented by medial marginal vein
(D) b & c both

19. Tributaries of great saphenous vein just before piercing into cribriform fascia are –
(A) superficial epigastric artery
(B) superficial circumflex artery
(C) superficial external pudendal vein
(D) all of the above

20. Tributaries of great saphenous vein just before opening in femoral vein –
(A) superficial epigastric artery
(B) superficial circumflex artery
(C) superficial external pudendal vein
(D) deep external pudendal vein

21. Number of valves present in great saphenous vein are –
(A) 5 to 10
(B) 10 to 20
(C) 16 to 24
(D) none of the above

22. Short saphenous vein starts from-
(A) lateral end of dorsal venous arch
(B) runs below the lateral malleolus
(C) accompanied by the sural nerve
(D) all of the above

23. Small saphenous vein has –
(A) 3-8 valves
(B) 7-13 valves
(C) 12-20 valves
(D) none of the above

24. Medial lymph nodes of superficial horizontal group drain-
(A) penis including prepuce & scrotum
(B) vulva & vagina below hymen
(C) perineum and lower part of anal canal below pectinate line
(D) all of the above

25. Lymphatic's from glans penis drain into-
(A) medial part of superficial lymph nodes
(B) lateral part of superficial lymph nodes
(C) deep inguinal lymph nodes
(D) all of the above

26. Saphenous opening is a gap in the-
(A) superficial fascia
(B) fascia lata
(C) iliotibial tract
(D) none of the above

27. Structures passing through saphenous opening are all except-
(A) great saphenous vein
(B) superficial epigastric & superficial external pudendal arteries
(C) superficial epigastric & superficial external pudendal veins
(D) branches of medial femoral cutaneous nerve

28. Iliotibial tract encloses-
(A) tensor fascia lata
(B) tensor fascia lata & gluteus maximus
(C) tensor fascia lata, gluteus maximus & minimus
(D) none of the above

29. Floor of femoral triangle is formed by-
(A) iliacus
(B) psoas major
(C) pectineus
(D) all of the above

30. Trunk of femoral nerve passes in a gap between-
(A) iliacus & psoas
(B) psoas & pectineus
(C) pectineus & adductor longus
(D) none of the above

31. Medial circumflex femoral vessels pass in a gap between-
(A) iliacus & psoas
(B) psoas & pectineus
(C) pectineus & adductor longus
(D) none of the above

32. Profunda femoral artery passes in a gap between-
(A) iliacus & psoas
(B) psoas & pectineus
(C) pectineus & adductor longus
(D) none of the above

33. Femoral artery in femoral triangle passes on all tendons except -
(A) adductor longus
(B) on psoas muscle
(C) on pectineus
(D) all of the above

34. In femoral triangle femoral artery anteriorly is crossed by-
(A) saphenous nerve
(B) ilio inguinal nerve
(C) medial femoral cutaneous nerve of thigh
(D) all of the above

35. In adductor canal femoral artery anteriorly is crossed by-
(A) saphenous nerve
(B) ilio inguinal nerve
(C) medial femoral cutaneous nerve of thigh
(D) all of the above

36. Spinous anastomosis at anterior superior iliac spine is formed by all except-
(A) superficial circumflex iliac artery superior gluteal
(B) superior gluteal artery
(C) superficial epigastric artery
(D) lateral circumflex femoral artery

37. Largest branch of femoral artery is-
(A) deep external pudendal artery
(B) profunda femoris artery
(C) descending genicular artery
(D) none of the above

38. Profunda femoris artery supplies –
(A) medial compartment of thigh
(B) anterior compartment of thigh
(C) posterior compartment of thigh
(D) all of the above

39. Branches of lateral circumflex femoral artery takes part in following anastomosis-
(A) spinous anastomosis
(B) cruciate anastomosis
(C) anastomosis around knee joint
(D) all of the above

40. Artery passing between anterior and posterior division of femoral nerve is-
(A) medial circumflex femoral artery
(B) lateral circumflex femoral artery
(C) profunda femoris artery
(D) none of the above

41. Perforating arteries are branches from-
(A) femoral artery
(B) profunda femoris artery
(C) medial circumflex femoral artery
(D) all of the above

42. Number of perforating arteries in thigh are-
(A) 3
(B) 4
(C) 5
(D) 6

43. All perforator arteries perforate –
(A) adductor longus
(B) adductor brevis
(C) adductor magnus
(D) all of the above

44. Adductor brevis is pierced by-
(A) 1st perforator
(B) 2nd perforator
(C) 3rd perforator
(D) 4th perforator

45. Perforator artery piercing both adductor brevis and magnus is-
(A) 1st perforator
(B) 2nd perforator
(C) 3rd perforator
(D) 4th perforator

46. Nutrient artery to femur is commonly given by-
(A) 1st perforator
(B) 2nd perforator
(C) 3rd perforator
(D) 4th perforator

47. Descending genicular artery is a branch from
(A) femoral artery
(B) profunda femoris artery
(C) lateral circumflex femoral artery
(D) all of the above

48. Descending genicular artery is given in-
(A) femoral triangle
(B) adductor canal
(C) popliteal fossa apex
(D) none of the above

49. Anterior layer of femoral sheath is derived from-
(A) external oblique aponeurosis
(B) internal oblique aponeurosis
(C) fascia transversalis
(D) fascia iliaca

50. Posterior layer of femoral sheath is derived from-
(A) external oblique aponeurosis
(B) internal oblique aponeurosis
(C) fascia transversalis
(D) fascia iliaca

51. Not a content of femoral sheath –
(A) femoral artery
(B) femoral vein
(C) femoral nerve
(D) lymph node

52. Lateral compartment of femoral sheath contains-
(A) femoral artery
(B) femoral vein
(C) femoral artery & femoral branch of genito femoral nerve
(D) femoral artery & femoral branch of ilio-inguinal nerve

53. True about boundaries of femoral ring is-
(A) anteriorly by inguinal ligament
(B) posteriorly by pectineus muscle
(C) medially by lacunar ligament
(D) all are true

54. Structures piercing femoral sheath are-
(A) superficial epigastric artery
(B) superficial circumflex iliac artery
(C) superficial external pudendal artery
(D) all of the above

55. Structures piercing femoral sheath are-
(A) great saphenous vein
(B) superficial epigastric artery
(C) femoral branch of genitofemoral nerve
(D) all of the above

56. Structures piercing femoral sheath on medial side are-
(A) great saphenous vein
(B) superficial epigastric artery
(C) femoral branch of genitofemoral nerve
(D) all of the above

57. Structures piercing femoral sheath on lateral side are-
(A) great saphenous vein
(B) superficial epigastric artery
(C) femoral branch of genitofemoral nerve
(D) all of the above

58. Structures piercing femoral sheath anteriorly are-
(A) great saphenous vein
(B) superficial epigastric artery
(C) femoral branch of genitofemoral nerve
(D) all of the above

59. Structures piercing femoral sheath anteriorly are-
(A) superficial epigastric artery
(B) superficial circumflex iliac artery
(C) superficial external pudendal artery
(D) all of the above

60. Largest branch of lumbar plexus is-
(A) obturator nerve
(B) sciatic nerve
(C) femoral nerve
(D) none of the above

61. Femoral nerve enters in thigh behind inguinal ligament –
(A) on psoas tendon
(B) between iliacus and psoas tendon
(C) on iliac tendon
(D) none of the above

62. Branches from trunk of femoral nerve are all except-
(A) to iliacus
(B) to pectineus
(C) to psoas
(D) vascular branches to femoral artery

63. Branches from anterior division of femoral nerve are-
(A) sartorius
(B) medial cutaneous femoral nerve
(C) intermediate femoral cutaneous nerve
(D) all of the above

64. Longest cutaneous nerve of body is-
(A) sural nerve
(B) saphenous nerve
(C) sciatic nerve
(D) posterior cutaneous nerve of thigh

65. Saphenous nerve arises from-
(A) trunk of femoral nerve
(B) anterior division of femoral nerve
(C) posterior division of femoral nerve
(D) all of the above

66. Hip joint is supplied by femoral nerve by articular branch from-
(A) nerve to sartorius
(B) nerve to rectus femoris
(C) separate branch trunk
(D) nerve to vastus medialis

67. Knee joint is supplied by femoral nerve by articular branch from-
(A) nerve to vastus lateralis
(B) nerve to vastus intermedius
(C) nerve to vastus medialis
(D) all of the above

68. Sartorius muscle is pierced by-
(A) intermediate femoral cutaneous nerve
(B) infrapatellar branch of saphenous nerve
(C) lateral femoral cutaneous nerve
(D) a and b

69. Action of sartorius at hip joint is-
(A) flexor, adductor & lateral rotator
(B) flexor, abductor & lateral rotator
(C) flexor, abductor & medial rotator
(D) extensor, adductor & lateral rotator

70. Action of sartorius at knee joint is-
(A) flexor & lateral rotator
(B) flexor & medial rotator
(C) extensor & medial rotator
(D) extensor& lateral rotator

71. Action of iliacus muscle at hip joint is-
(A) flexor & lateral rotator
(B) flexor & medial rotator
(C) extensor & medial rotator
(D) extensor& lateral rotator

72. Iliacus is supplied by trunk of femoral nerve by-
(A) L2L3L4 roots
(B) L2L3 roots
(C) L3L4 roots
(D) none of the above

73. Psoas major muscle is supplied by -
(A) L2L3L4 roots of femoral nerve
(B) L2L3 roots of lumbar plexus
(C) L3L4 roots of lumbar plexus
(D) none of the above

74. Pectineus muscle is supplied by-
(A) femoral nerve
(B) obturator nerve
(C) both a & b
(D) none of the above

75. Boundaries of adductor canal are-
(A) floor-adductor longus & magnus
(B) roof- sartorius
(C) laterally-vastus medially
(D) all of the above

76. Sub sartorial plexus is formed by all except-
(A) saphenous nerve
(B) intermediate femoral cutaneous nerve
(C) obturator nerve
(D) medial femoral cutaneous nerve

77. Contents of Hunter's canal are-
(A) femoral artery
(B) femoral vein
(C) saphenous nerve
(D) all of the above

78. Contents of Hunter's canal are-
(A) saphenous nerve
(B) posterior division of obturator nerve
(C) nerve to vastus medialis
(D) all of the above

79. Largest muscle of the body is-
(A) gluteus maximus
(B) quadriceps femoris
(C) rectus femoris
(D) external oblique of abdomen

80. Rectus femoris muscle is-
(A) unipinnate
(B) bipinnate
(C) multipinnate
(D) none of the above

Answersheet

1. **D**	2. **B**	3. **A**	4. **B**	5. **B**	6. **B**	7. **D**	8. **B**	9. **A**	10. **B**
11. **B**	12. **D**	13. **D**	14. **D**	15. **B**	16. **C**	17. **B**	18. **D**	19. **D**	20. **D**
21. **B**	22. **D**	23. **B**	24. **D**	25. **C**	26. **B**	27. **C**	28. **B**	29. **D**	30. **A**
31. **B**	32. **C**	33. **D**	34. **C**	35. **A**	36. **C**	37. **B**	38. **D**	39. **D**	40. **B**
41. **B**	42. **B**	43. **C**	44. **B**	45. **B**	46. **B**	47. **A**	48. **B**	49. **C**	50. **D**
51. **C**	52. **C**	53. **D**	54. **D**	55. **D**	56. **A**	57. **C**	58. **B**	59. **D**	60. **C**
61. **B**	62. **C**	63. **D**	64. **B**	65. **C**	66. **B**	67. **D**	68. **D**	69. **B**	70. **B**
71. **B**	72. **B**	73. **B**	74. **C**	75. **D**	76. **B**	77. **D**	78. **D**	79. **B**	80. **B**

Chapter **12**

Posterior Compartment of Thigh and Popliteal Fossa

1. All are true about hamstrings-
(A) take origin from ischeal tuberosity
(B) inserted in any of leg bones
(C) supplied by sciatic nerve
(D) all of the above

2. All are true about nerve supply of true hamstrings-
(A) supplied by sciatic nerve
(B) by tibial division of sciatic nerve
(C) by common peroneal division of sciatic nerve
(D) all of the above

3. Actions of hamstrings is-
(A) extensor at hip and extensor at knee joint
(B) extensor at hip and flexor at knee joint
(C) flexor at hip and extensor at knee joint
(D) flexor at hip and flexor at knee joint

4. True hamstring muscle is-
(A) adductor magnus
(B) biceps femoris
(C) semitendinosus
(D) none of the above

5. True hamstring muscle is-
(A) adductor magnus
(B) biceps femoris
(C) semimembranosus
(D) none of the above

6. Modified hamstring muscle is-
(A) adductor magnus
(B) biceps femoris short head
(C) long head of biceps femoris
(D) semitendinosus

7. Modified hamstring muscle is-
(A) adductor head of adductor magnus
(B) biceps femoris short head
(C) ischeal head of adductor magnus
(D) semimembranosus

8. Sacrotuberous ligament is modified attachment of-
(A) hamstring part of adductor magnus
(B) short head of biceps
(C) long head of biceps
(D) none of the above

9. Tibial collateral ligament is modified attachment of-
(A) adductor magnus
(B) adductor brevis
(C) adductor longus
(D) semitendinosus

10. Oblique popliteal ligament is derivative of-
(A) semitendinosus
(B) semimembranosus
(C) biceps femoris
(D) adductor magnus

11. Short head of biceps femoris -
(A) supplied by common peroneal nerve
(B) attached to femur
(C) morphologically represents extensor compartment
(D) all of the above

12. Medial rotators at knee joint –
(A) semitendinosus & biceps femoris
(B) semimembranosus & semimembranosus
(C) adductor magnus & biceps femoris
(D) semimembranosus & biceps femoris

13. Lateral rotators at knee joint –
(A) semitendinosus
(B) biceps femoris
(C) adductor magnus & biceps femoris
(D) semimembranosus & biceps femoris

14. Supero-lateral boundary of popliteal fossa is-
(A) semimembranosus & semitendinosus
(B) biceps femoris
(C) plantaris & lateral head of gastrocnemius
(D) medial head of gastrocnemius

15. Supero-medial boundary of popliteal fossa is-
(A) semimembranosus & semitendinosus
(B) biceps femoris
(C) plantaris & lateral head of gastrocnemius
(D) medial head of gastrocnemius

16. Infero-lateral boundary of popliteal fossa is-
(A) semimembranosus & semitendinosus
(B) biceps femoris
(C) plantaris & lateral head of gastrocnemius
(D) medial head of gastrocnemius

17. Infero-medial boundary of popliteal fossa is-
(A) semimembranosus & semitendinosus
(B) biceps femoris
(C) plantaris & lateral head of gastrocnemius
(D) medial head of gastrocnemius

18. Floor of popliteal fossa is formed by-
(A) popliteal surface of femur & tibia
(B) oblique popliteal ligament
(C) fascia covering popliteus
(D) all of the above

19. Floor of the popliteal fossa is pierced by-
(A) middle genicular vessels
(B) middle genicular nerve
(C) genicular branch of obturator nerve
(D) all of the above

20. Roof of popliteal fossa is pierced by-
(A) small saphenous vein & post cut n of thigh
(B) great saphenous vein & post cut n of thigh
(C) saphenous nerve & small saphenous nerve
(D) none of the above

21. All are contents of popliteal fossa except-
(A) popliteal artery
(B) popliteal vein
(C) small saphenous vein
(D) popliteal lymph nodes

22. All are contents of popliteal fossa except-
(A) popliteal artery
(B) popliteal vein
(C) small saphenous vein
(D) popliteal lymph nodes

23. Nerves present in popliteal fossa are-
(A) tibial nerve
(B) common peroneal nerve
(C) posterior cutaneous nerve of thigh
(D) all of the above

24. True about posterior cutaneous nerve of thigh is-
(A) present in roof
(B) pierces floor of popliteal fossa
(C) is a content of popliteal fossa
(D) all of the above

25. Tibial nerve crosses popliteal artery and vein-
(A) from medial to lateral
(B) from lateral to medial
(C) from deep to superficial
(D) none of the above

26. Artery piercing the oblique popliteal ligament is-
(A) superior medial genicular artery
(B) middle genicular artery
(C) inferior medial genicular artery
(D) all of the above

27. Medial popliteal nerve is-
(A) sciatic nerve
(B) tibial nerve
(C) common peroneal nerve
(D) none of the above

28. Lateral popliteal nerve is-
(A) sciatic nerve
(B) tibial nerve
(C) common peroneal nerve
(D) none of the above

29. Larger terminal branch of sciatic nerve is-
(A) common peroneal nerve
(B) tibial nerve
(C) both are equal
(D) all of the above

30. True about tibial nerve relations in popliteal fossa is-
(A) tibial nerve is lateral to popliteal vessels in upper part
(B) tibial nerve is medial to popliteal vessels in lower part
(C) tibial nerve is posterior to popliteal vessels in middle part
(D) all of the above

31. Nerve to popliteus supplies-
(A) superior & inferior tibiofibular joints
(B) tibialis posterior
(C) tibia bone
(D) all of the above

32. Articular branches from common peroneal nerve are all except-
(A) superior lateral genicular
(B) inferior lateral genicular
(C) recurrent genicular
(D) middle genicular

33. Articular branches from tibial nerve are all except-
(A) superior medial genicular
(B) inferior medial genicular
(C) recurrent genicular
(D) middle genicular

34. Oblique popliteal ligament is pierced by-
(A) superior lateral genicular
(B) inferior medial genicular
(C) recurrent genicular
(D) middle genicular

35. Sural nerve is a branch from-
(A) sciatic nerve
(B) tibial nerve
(C) common peroneal nerve
(D) nerve to popliteus

36. Tibialis anterior muscle is pierced by-
(A) inferior lateral genicular nerve
(B) recurrent genicular nerve
(C) superior lateral genicular nerve
(D) none of the above

37. Common peroneal nerve divides into terminal branches –
(A) in popliteal fossa
(B) at the neck of fibula
(C) in the anterior compartment of leg
(D) none of the above

38. Foot drop may occur due to injury of-
(A) femoral nerve
(B) obturator nerve
(C) sciatic nerve
(D) all of the above

39. Foot drop may occur due to injury of-
(A) common peroneal nerve
(B) deep peroneal nerve
(C) sciatic nerve
(D) all of the above

40. Foot drop may occur due to injury of all except-
(A) common peroneal nerve
(B) deep peroneal nerve
(C) superficial peroneal nerve
(D) sciatic nerve

41. Foot drop may occur due to-
(A) bumper fracture
(B) fracture neck fibula
(C) pressure of plaster cast of leg
(D) all of the above

42. Deepest structure in the popliteal fossa is-
(A) tibial nerve
(B) popliteal artery
(C) popliteal vein
(D) common peroneal nerve

Answersheet

1. **D**	2. **B**	3. **B**	4. **C**	5. **C**	6. **C**	7. **C**	8. **C**	9. **A**	10. **B**
11. **D**	12. **B**	13. **B**	14. **B**	15. **A**	16. **C**	17. **D**	18. **D**	19. **D**	20. **A**
21. **C**	22. **C**	23. **D**	24. **D**	25. **B**	26. **B**	27. **B**	28. **C**	29. **B**	30. **D**
31. **D**	32. **D**	33. **C**	34. **D**	35. **B**	36. **B**	37. **B**	38. **C**	39. **D**	40. **C**
41. **D**	42. **B**								

Chapter **13**

Medial Compartment of Thigh

1. Medial compartment of thigh is represented in upper limb as-

(A) biceps brachii

(B) brachialis

(C) coracobrachialis

(D) all of the above

2. Muscles of medial compartment are adductors except-

(A) adductor longus

(B) adductor magnus

(C) obturator internus

(D) obturator externus

3. Adductor magnus is supplied by-

(A) femoral nerve & obturator nerve

(B) obturator nerve & common peroneal nerve

(C) tibial nerve & obturator nerve

(D) none of the above

4. Pectineus muscle is supplied by-

(A) femoral nerve & obturator nerve

(B) obturator nerve & common peroneal nerve

(C) tibial nerve & obturator nerve

(D) none of the above

5. All are true about pectineus muscle except-

(A) quadrangular muscle

(B) lies in between psoas & adductor longus

(C) attached to greater trochanter

(D) all are true

6. True about adductor longus is all except-

(A) adductor of thigh at hip joint

(B) medial rotator of thigh at hip joint

(C) supplied by anterior div of obturator nerve

(D) supplied by posterior div of obturator nerve

7. Rider's bone a sesamoid bone may develop in the tendon of-

(A) adductor longus

(B) adductor brevis

(C) adductor magnus

(D) none of the above

8. All are actions of adductor magnus except-

(A) adduction of thigh at hip joint

(B) medial rotation of thigh

(C) flexor at hip joint

(D) extensor at hip joint

9. Muscle of adductor compartment not attached at femur is-
(A) adductor magnus
(B) pectineus
(C) gracilis
(D) adductor brevis

10. All are actions of gracilis except-
(A) adduction of thigh
(B) medial rotation of thigh
(C) flexor of leg at knee
(D) flexor of thigh at hip

11. Action of obturator externus is-
(A) adduction of thigh
(B) medial rotation of thigh
(C) flexor of leg at knee
(D) lateral rotation of thigh at hip

12. Root value of obturator nerve is-
(A) L2L3L4
(B) dorsal division of L2L3L4
(C) ventral division of L2L3L4
(D) all of the above

13. Anterior division of obturator nerve supplies all except-
(A) pectineus
(B) adductor longus
(C) obturator externus
(D) gracilis

14. Posterior division of obturator nerve supplies all except-
(A) adductor longus
(B) adductor brevis
(C) adductor magnus
(D) obturator externus

15. Obturator externus is pierced by-
(A) obturator nerve
(B) anterior division of obturator nerve
(C) posterior division of obturator nerve
(D) all of the above

16. Hip joint is supplied by-
(A) obturator nerve
(B) anterior division of obturator nerve
(C) posterior division of obturator nerve
(D) all of the above

17. Knee joint is supplied by-
(A) obturator nerve
(B) anterior division of obturator nerve
(C) posterior division of obturator nerve
(D) all of the above

18. True about accessory obturator nerve is all except-
(A) root value is L2L3
(B) root value is L3L4
(C) supplies pectineus muscle
(D) supplies hip joint

19. Obturator canal gives passage to-
(A) obturator nerve
(B) obturator artery
(C) both a & b
(D) none of the above

20. Adductor magnus muscle is pierced by-
(A) 1st perforator artery
(B) 2nd perforator artery
(C) 3rd perforator artery
(D) 4th perforator artery

21. Largest branch of profunda femoris artery is-
(A) medial circumflex femoral artery
(B) lateral circumflex femoral artery
(C) perforating arteries
(D) none of the above

22. Largest muscle of adductor compartment of thigh is-
(A) adductor longus
(B) adductor brevis
(C) adductor magnus
(D) obturator externus

23. Part of guy ropes are all except-
(A) sartorius
(B) semi membranosus
(C) semi tendeniosus
(D) gracilis

24. Action of gracilis muscle are all except-
(A) adductor at hip
(B) flexion at hip
(C) flexion at knee
(D) medial rotator at knee

25. Hip joint is supplied by obturator nerve by-
(A) trunk
(B) anterior division
(C) posterior division
(D) all of the above

26. Knee joint is supplied by obturator nerve by-
(A) trunk
(B) anterior division
(C) posterior division
(D) all of the above

27. Obturator artery is a branch from-
(A) internal iliac artery
(B) anterior division of internal iliac artery
(C) posterior division of internal iliac artery
(D) none of the above

28. Name custodian of virginity is given to-
(A) adductor longus
(B) gracilis
(C) adductor brevis
(D) adductor magnus

29. Muscles in superficial stratum in medial compartment of thigh are all except-
(A) pectineus
(B) adductor longus
(C) obturator externus
(D) gracilis

30. Rider's muscle is-
(A) adductor longus
(B) adductor brevis
(C) adductor magnus
(D) all of the above

31. Anterior relation of pectineus in femoral triangle is-
(A) femoral nerve
(B) femoral artery
(C) obturator nerve
(D) great saphenous vein

32. Artery present in a gap between pectineus & adductor longus is-
(A) femoral artery
(B) profunda femoris artery
(C) femoral vein
(D) obturator nerve

33. Rider's bone develops as sesamoid bone in the tendon of-
(A) adductor longus
(B) adductor brevis
(C) adductor magnus
(D) all of the above

34. Adductor longus near its origin, anteriorly is crossed by-
(A) profunda femoris artery
(B) spermatic cord in male
(C) obturator nerve
(D) none of the above

35. Posterior relations of adductor longus is-
(A) profunda femoris artery
(B) anterior branch of obturator nerve
(C) adductor brevis muscle
(D) all of the above

36. Action of gracilis is-
(A) flexion of leg
(B) medial rotation of thigh
(C) adduction of thigh
(D) all of the above

Answersheet

1. **C**	2. **D**	3. **C**	4. **A**	5. **C**	6. **D**	7. **A**	8. **C**	9. **C**	10. **D**
11. **D**	12. **C**	13. **C**	14. **A**	15. **C**	16. **B**	17. **C**	18. **A**	19. **C**	20. **D**
21. **B**	22. **C**	23. **B**	24. **B**	25. **B**	26. **C**	27. **B**	28. **B**	29. **C**	30. **D**
31. **B**	32. **B**	33. **A**	34. **B**	35. **D**	36. **D**				

Chapter **14**

Leg

1. Superficial flexor muscles of posterior compartment are-
(A) plantaris
(B) gastrocnemius
(C) soleus
(D) all of the above

2. Tendo calcaneus is formed by-
(A) medial head of gastrocnemius
(B) lateral head of gastrocnemius
(C) soleus
(D) all of the above

3. Morphologically soleus corresponds to-
(A) palmaris longus of forearm
(B) flexor digitorum superficialis of forearm
(C) flexor digitorum profundus of forearm
(D) none of the above

4. Detached portion of soleus is represented by-
(A) first lumbrical
(B) flexor hallucis brevis
(C) flexor digitorum brevis
(D) none of the above

5. Muscle called as peripheral heart is-
(A) gastrocnemius
(B) soleus
(C) plantaris
(D) tibialis posterior

6. All are bipinnate muscles except-
(A) flexor digitorum longus
(B) gastrocnemius
(C) tibialis posterior
(D) flexor hallucis longus

7. Triceps surae muscle is composed of-
(A) gastrocnemius & popliteus
(B) gastrocnemius & soleus
(C) gastrocnemius, popliteus & plantaris
(D) gastrocnemius , popliteus &soleus

8. Soleus is-
(A) unipinnate
(B) bipinnate
(C) multipinnate
(D) none of the above

9. Tendon passing through groove between medial & posterior tubercle of talus is-
(A) flexor digitorum longus
(B) flexor hallucis longus
(C) tibialis posterior
(D) none of the above

10. Action of tibialis posterior is-
(A) maintains medial longitudenal arch of foot
(B) plantar flexion at ankle
(C) inverter & adductor of forefoot
(D) all of the above

11. Action of flexor hallucis longus is-
(A) maintains medial longitudenal arch of foot
(B) plantar flexion at great toe
(C) plantar flexion at ankle
(D) all of the above

12. Posterior tibial artery arises from popliteal artery at-
(A) upper border of popliteus
(B) lower border of popliteus
(C) neck of fibula
(D) popliteal fossa

13. In upper half of leg tibial nerve is-
(A) anterior to posterior tibial artery
(B) lateral to posterior tibial artery
(C) medial to posterior tibial artery
(D) posterior to posterior tibial artery

14. In lower half of leg tibial nerve is-
(A) anterior to posterior tibial artery
(B) lateral to posterior tibial artery
(C) medial to posterior tibial artery
(D) posterior to posterior tibial artery

15. Most medial structure in flexor retinaculum posterior to ankle is-
(A) tibialis posterior
(B) flexor digitorum longus
(C) posterior tibial artery
(D) flexor hallucis longus tendon

16. Most lateral structure in flexor retinaculum posterior to ankle is-
(A) tibialis posterior
(B) flexor digitorum longus
(C) posterior tibial artery
(D) flexor hallucis longus tendon

17. Tibialis anterior muscle is-
(A) unipinnate
(B) bipinnate
(C) multipinnate
(D) none of the above

18. Action of tibialis anterior is-
(A) dorsi flexor of foot at ankle joint
(B) invertor of foot
(C) maintains medial longitudenal arch of foot
(D) all of the above

19. Extensor hallucis longus is –
(A) unipinnate
(B) bipinnate
(C) multipinnate
(D) none of the above

20. Peroneus longus is –
(A) unipinnate
(B) bipinnate
(C) multipinnate
(D) none of the above

21. Peroneus tertitus is supplied by-
(A) common peroneal nerve
(B) deep peroneal nerve
(C) superficial peroneal nerve
(D) none of the above

22. Peroneus longus is supplied by-
(A) common peroneal nerve
(B) deep peroneal nerve
(C) superficial peroneal nerve
(D) none of the above

23. Small saphenous vein starts from-
(A) lateral side of dorsal venous arch
(B) medial side of dorsal venous arch
(C) both a & b
(D) none of the above

24. Great saphenous vein starts from-
(A) lateral side of dorsal venous arch
(B) medial side of dorsal venous arch
(C) both a & b
(D) none of the above

25. Intrinsic muscle on the dorsum of foot is-
(A) tibialis anterior
(B) extensor digitorum brevis
(C) peroneus tertius
(D) none of the above

26. Extensor digitorum brevis is supplied by-
(A) common peroneal nerve
(B) deep peroneal nerve
(C) superficial peroneal nerve
(D) none of the above

27. All muscles of anterior compartment arise from fibula except-
(A) tibialis anterior
(B) extensor digitorum longus
(C) extensor hallucis longus
(D) peroneus tertius

28. Musculocutaneous nerve of lower limb is-
(A) sciatic nerve
(B) common peroneal nerve
(C) deep peroneal nerve
(D) superficial peroneal nerve

29. Nervous hesitant of lower limb is-
(A) sciatic nerve
(B) common peroneal nerve
(C) deep peroneal nerve
(D) superficial peroneal nerve

30. Peroneus longus is inserted at-
(A) tubercle at the base of fifth metatarsal
(B) base of first meta tarsal & medial cuneiform
(C) both a & c
(D) none of the above

31. Peroneus brevis is inserted at-
(A) tubercle at the base of fifth metatarsal
(B) base of first meta tarsal & medial cuneiform
(C) both a & c
(D) none of the above

32. Action of peroneus longus-
(A) evertor of foot
(B) maintains lateral longitudenal arch of foot
(C) maintains transverse arch of foot
(D) all of the above

33. Most commonly injured nerve of lower limb -
(A) femoral nerve
(B) obturator nerve
(C) common peroneal nerve
(D) tibial nerve

34. All are part of guy ropes except-
(A) gracilis
(B) sartorius
(C) semitendinosus
(D) semimembranosus

35. All are superficial muscles of back of thigh except-
(A) gastrocnemius
(B) popliteus
(C) soleus
(D) plantaris

36. Largest nutrient artery of body is-
(A) nutrient artery of humerus
(B) nutrient artery of femur
(C) nutrient artery of tibia
(D) nutrient artery of fibula

37. Largest nutrient artery of body is a branch of-
(A) nutrient artery from brachial artery
(B) nutrient artery from femoral artery
(C) nutrient artery from posterior tibial artery
(D) nutrient artery from radial artery

38. Peroneus tertitus is regarded as detached part of –
(A) tibialis anterior
(B) extensor digitorum longus
(C) extensor digitorum brevis
(D) extensor hallucis longus

39. Peroneus longus is responsible for maintenance of-
(A) medial longitudinal arch of foot
(B) lateral longitudinal arch of foot
(C) transverse arch of foot
(D) all of the above

40. Tendon passing deep to sustentaculum tali is-
(A) tibialis posterior
(B) flexor hallucis longus
(C) extensor hallucis longus
(D) peroneus longus

41. Largest branch of posterior tibial artery is-
(A) circumflex fibular artery
(B) peroneal artery
(C) calcaneal branch
(D) malleolar branch

42. Deep peroneal nerve begins in the substance of –
(A) peroneus longus
(B) peroneus brevis
(C) peroneus tertitus
(D) none of the above

43. Nervus hesitans is the name given to-
(A) common peroneal nerve
(B) deep peroneal nerve
(C) superficial peroneal nerve
(D) none of the above

44. Cuboid bone is grooved by tendon of-
(A) peroneus longus
(B) peroneus brevis
(C) peroneus tertitus
(D) tibialis posterior

45. Largest compartment of the leg is-
(A) anterior
(B) posterior
(C) lateral
(D) none of the above

46. Muscle present in superficial part of posterior compartment of leg are all except-
(A) gastrocnemius
(B) tibialis posterior
(C) soleus
(D) plantaris

47. Deepest placed muscle in posterior compartment of leg is-

(A) gastrocnemius
(B) tibialis posterior
(C) soleus
(D) popliteus

48. In tennis leg there is detachment and pain at-

(A) medial head of gastrocnemius
(B) lateral head of gastrocnemius
(C) soleus
(D) plantaris

Answersheet

1. **D**	2. **D**	3. **B**	4. **C**	5. **B**	6. **B**	7. **B**	8. **C**	9. **B**	10. **D**
11. **D**	12. **B**	13. **C**	14. **B**	15. **A**	16. **D**	17. **C**	18. **D**	19. **A**	20. **B**
21. **B**	22. **C**	23. **A**	24. **B**	25. **B**	26. **B**	27. **A**	28. **D**	29. **C**	30. **B**
31. **A**	32. **D**	33. **C**	34. **D**	35. **B**	36. **C**	37. **C**	38. **B**	39. **D**	40. **B**
41. **B**	42. **A**	43. **B**	44. **A**	45. **B**	46. **B**	47. **B**	48. **A**		

Chapter 15

Foot

1. Area where fibro- fatty tissue is more abundant:
   (A) Posterior tubercle of calcaneus
   (B) Metatarsals head
   (C) Pulp of terminal digits
   (D) All are the sites of accumulation

2. Over weight bearing area of heel, skin is supplied by:
   (A) Calcaneal branch of tibial nerve
   (B) Sural nerve
   (C) Saphenous nerve
   (D) Medial planter nerve

3. Medial part of sole including planter surface of medial three and half toes are supplied by:
   (A) Sural nerve
   (B) Medial planter nerve
   (C) Saphenous nerve
   (D) Calcaneal branch of tibial nerve

4. First interdigital cleft of foot is supplied by:
   (A) Sural nerve
   (B) Deep peroneal nerve
   (C) Saphenous nerve
   (D) Medial planter nerve

5. True statement regarding planter aponeurosis is/are:
   (A) Composed of compact bundle of collagen fibres
   (B) Consists of three parts
   (C) Central part covers flexor digitorum brevis
   (D) All are true

6. True statement regarding central part of planter aponeurosis is/ are:
   (A) Attached to medial tubercle of calcaneus
   (B) Anterior part split in four band
   (C) Represent continuation of soleus tendon
   (D) All are true

7. Superficial stratum of central part is attached to:
   (A) Dermis by skin ligaments
   (B) Bled with superficial transvers metatarsal ligament
   (C) Both are true
   (D) None of above

8. Deep stratum of central part is attached to:

(A) Fibrous flexor sheath

(B) Embrace to flexor tendons

(C) Deep transvers metatarsal ligament

(D) All are true

9. Medial intermuscular septum is characterized by:

(A) Subdivided into three part

(B) Distal segment split to enclose flexor hallucis longus tendon

(C) Attached to first metatarsal bone

(D) All are true

10. Lateral intermuscular septum is characterized by:

(A) Subdivided into two parts

(B) Attached to fifth metatarsal bone

(C) Both are true

(D) None of above

11. All are true statement regarding medial part of planter aponeurosis except:

(A) Covers abductor hallucis

(B) Continuous posteriorly with flexor retinaculum

(C) Medially continue with deep fascia of dorsum of foot

(D) Lateral part of it thickened and form fibrous band

12. Functions of planter aponeurosis is / are:

(A) Maintains longitudinal arches

(B) Provide origin to superficial groups of planter muscle

(C) Protect planter nerve and vessels from compression

(D) All are true

13. All are muscle of first layer of sole except:

(A) Abductor halluces

(B) Flexor digitorum brevis

(C) Flexor digitorum accessories

(D) Abductor digiti minimi

14. All are origin point for abductor halluces muscle except:

(A) Posterior tubercle of calcaneus

(B) Planter aponeurosis

(C) Flexor retinaculum

(D) Medial intermuscular septum

15. True statement regarding abductor halluces muscle is/ are:

(A) Takes origin from posterior tubercle of calcaneus

(B) Gets inserted on lateral side of base of proximal phalanx of great toe

(C) Supplied by medial planter nerve

(D) All are true

16. True statement regarding flexor digitorum brevis is/ are:

(A) Lies deep to central part of planter aponeurosis

(B) Mode of insertion is identical with flexor digitorum profundus of hand

(C) Produce dorsi flexion of lateral four toes

(D) All are true

17. All are origin points of abductor digiti minimi except:

(A) Medial tubercle of calcaneus

(B) Lateral tubercle of calcaneus

(C) Flexor retinaculum

(D) Planter aponeurosis

18. Wood's muscle is:
(A) Sometime medial fibers of abductor digiti minimi gets inserted to fifth metatarsal bone
(B) Supplied by medial planter nerve
(C) Both are true
(D) None of above

19. All are muscle of second layer of sole except:
(A) Tendon of flexor hallucis longus
(B) Flexor digitorum brevis
(C) Four lumbricals
(D) Flexor digitorum accessorius

20. Tendon passes from undersurface of sustentaculum tali of calcaneus:
(A) Flexor hallucis longus
(B) Tibialis anterior
(C) Peroneus longus
(D) Extensor hallucis longus

21. True statement regarding flexor digitorum longus is /are:
(A) Present above flexor retinaculum in sole
(B) Passes forward and medially
(C) Crossed superficial to tendon of flexor hallucis longus
(D) All of above are true

22. All are true statement regarding flexor digitorum accessories except:
(A) It has two heads
(B) Both head separated by long planter ligament
(C) Inserted into lateral side of common tendon of flexor digitorum longus
(D) Supplied by trunk of medial planter nerve

23. True statement regarding lumbricals of foot is /are:
(A) Numbered from medial to lateral side
(B) Takes origin from tendons of flexor digitorum brevis
(C) All are bipennate
(D) All are true

24. Lumbricals of foot get inserted to:
(A) On medial side of base of proximal phalanx of corresponding lateral four toes
(B) Dorsal surface of base of middle phalanx of lateral four toes
(C) Dorsal surface of base of terminal phalanx of lateral four toes
(D) All are insertion points of lumbricals

25. All are true statement regarding lumbricals except:
(A) May cause planter flexion at metatarso- phalangeal joint and dorsi flexion at interphalangeal joint
(B) Increase grip of metatarsal heads on ground for forward thrust of body
(C) All are supplied by lateral planter nerve
(D) Prevent buckling of toes during walking

26. All are muscle of third layer of sole except:
(A) Flexor hallucis brevis
(B) Abductor hallucis
(C) Adductor hallucis
(D) Flexor digiti minimi brevis

27. True statement regarding flexor hallucis brevis muscle is / are:

(A) Tendon of flexor hallucis longus lodge in groove of brevis muscle

(B) Supplied by lateral planter muscle

(C) Produce dorsi flexion of metatarso-phalangeal joint of great toe

(D) All are true

28. Regarding insertion of flexor hallucis brevis true statement is:

(A) Medial tendon is inserted in common with tendon of abductor hallucis

(B) Lateral tendon is inserted in common with adductor hallucis

(C) Both are true

(D) None of above

29. Oblique head of adductor hallucis arises from:

(A) Base of second to fourth metatarsal bones

(B) Sheath of peroneus longus muscle

(C) Both are true

(D) None of above

30. True statement regarding transvers head of adductor hallucis muscle is/ are:

(A) Has no bony origin

(B) Arises from deep transverse metatarsal ligaments

(C) From planter metatarso-phalangeal ligaments of third to fifth toes

(D) All are true

31. Structure present deep to oblique head of adductor hallucis:

(A) Planter arterial arch

(B) Deep branch of lateral planter nerve

(C) Both are present

(D) None of above

32. Adductor hallucis is supplied by:

(A) Deep branch of lateral planter nerve

(B) Nerve to second lumbrical

(C) Medial planter nerve

(D) From superficial branch of lateral planter nerve

33. Structure present deep to transvers head of adductor hallucis:

(A) Deep branch of lateral planter nerve

(B) Nerve to second lumbrical

(C) Medial planter nerve

(D) Planter arterial arch

34. All are true statement regarding flexor digiti minimi brevis except:

(A) Arises from planter surface of base of fifth metatarsal bone

(B) Inserted on lateral side base of proximal phalanx of little toe

(C) Supplied by deep branch of lateral planter nerve

(D) Originated from sheath of peroneus longus

35. True statement regarding dorsal interossei is /are:

(A) They are three in number

(B) Abductors of toes

(C) Numbered from lateral to medial side

(D) All are true

36. True statement regarding dorsal interossei is / are:

(A) All are bipennate in nature

(B) Dorsal pedis artery transmit between two heads of first dorsal interosseous

(C) Proximal perforating arteries passes between two heads of other interosseous

(D) All are true

37. True statement regarding planter interossei is / are:
(A) They are four in number
(B) All are bipennate
(C) Act as adductor of lateral three toes
(D) All are true

38. All are true statement regarding planter interossei except:
(A) Arises from medial side of planter surface of shaft of lateral three metatarsal bones
(B) Inserted on medial side of base of proximal phalanx of corresponding toe
(C) Act as adductor of lateral three toe
(D) All are supplied by deep branch of lateral planter nerve

39. All are the sites of attachment of tibialis posterior muscle except:
(A) Tuberosity of navicular bone
(B) Base of fifth metatarsal bone
(C) Cuboid bone
(D) Base of third metatarsal bone

40. Medial planter nerve supply all muscles except:
(A) Abductor hallucis
(B) Flexor digitorum longus
(C) Flexor hallucis brevis
(D) First lumbrical

41. Trunk of lateral planter nerve supply the muscle:
(A) Abductor digiti minimi
(B) Flexor digitorum brevis
(C) Both are supplied by
(D) None of above

42. All are muscles supplied by superficial branch of lateral planter nerve:
(A) Flexor digiti minimi brevis
(B) Fourth dorsal interossei
(C) Oblique head of adductor hallucis
(D) Third planter interossei

43. Muscle supplied by deep branch of lateral planter nerve is / are:
(A) First lumbrical
(B) Both heads of adductor hallucis
(C) Flexor digiti minimi brevis
(D) Third planter interossei

44. All are muscle supplied by deep branch of lateral planter nerve except:
(A) Second to fourth lumbricals
(B) Medial two planter interossei
(C) Fourth dorsal interossei
(D) Adductor hallucis

Answersheet

1. **D**	2. **A**	3. **B**	4. **B**	5. **D**	6. **A**	7. **C**	8. **D**	9. **D**	10. **B**
11. **D**	12. **D**	13. **C**	14. **A**	15. **C**	16. **A**	17. **C**	18. **A**	19. **B**	20. **A**
21. **C**	22. **D**	23. **A**	24. **D**	25. **C**	26. **B**	27. **A**	28. **C**	29. **C**	30. **D**
31. **C**	32. **A**	33. **B**	34. **C**	35. **B**	36. **D**	37. **C**	38. **D**	39. **B**	40. **B**
41. **A**	42. **C**	43. **B**	44. **C**						

Chapter 16

Joints of Lower Limb

1. True statement regarding head of femur is:
   (A) It is oval in shape
   (B) Resemble about 2/3 of a sphere.
   (C) All part of head is articular
   (D) None of above

2. True statement regarding acetabulum is/ are:
   (A) It is a complete socket
   (B) Margins give attachment to labrum in its whole length
   (C) Site where ilium, ischium and pubis meet, separated by a triradiate Y shaped cartilage
   (D) All of above

3. All are true regarding acetabulum except:
   (A) It has a notch
   (B) Postero – superior part of articular surface is thickest
   (C) Floor of it also articular
   (D) Notch gives attachment to transvers acetabular ligament

4. Acetabular fat is characterized by:
   (A) Remain in liquid condition at body temperature
   (B) It is extracapsular
   (C) It is intra synovial
   (D) All of above

5. All are true statement regarding capsular ligament of hip joint except:
   (A) Fibres are spirally arranged and taut in extension
   (B) Attached close to acetabular margins extending 5 to 6 mm above the labrum
   (C) Blend with anterior surface of labrum in front
   (D) None of above

6. Capsular ligament of hip joint is characterized by:
   (A) It covers anterior surface of femoral neck completely
   (B) It is attached along intertrochanteric line
   (C) Infero- medial part of it is weakest
   (D) All of above

7. Acetabular labrum is characterized by:
   (A) It is hyline cartilaginous rim attached to acetabular margins
   (B) Square in cross section
   (C) Not only deepen the socket but grasps femoral head tightly
   (D) None of above

8. All are true regarding ligament of the head of femur except:

(A) Triangular in shape
(B) Stretched in abduction of semiflexed hip
(C) Blends with the transvers acetabular ligament
(D) Apex is attached to the fovea of the femoral head

9. True statement regarding ligament of the head of femur is/ are:

(A) Increase the stability of joints
(B) Convey blood vessels to the head of femur
(C) Relaxed in adduction of semiflexed hip
(D) All of above

10. True statement regarding pubo- femoral ligament is/ are:

(A) Covers the infero- medial part of capsule
(B) Attached close to acetabular margin to the iliopubic eminence and obturator crest
(C) Blends with capsule deep to medial band of ilio- femoral ligament
(D) All of above

11. All are true regarding ilio- femoral ligament except:

(A) Also called as ligament of Bigelow
(B) Inverted Y shaped ligament
(C) Apex attach on anterior superior iliac spine
(D) Medial band attach to lower part of intertrochentric line

12. True statement regarding ilio- femoral ligament is:

(A) Prevent hyperflexion of hip joint
(B) Strengthen medial part of hip capsule
(C) Lateral band attach to intertrochentric crest
(D) Intermediate strata is pierced by ascending branch of lateral circumflex femoral artery

13. All are true statement regarding flexion of hip joint except:

(A) Flexion of hip with extended knee joint is limited to about 90°- 100°
(B) Flexion makes the joint closed packed condition and the capsule is taut
(C) 120° flexion is possible when knee is flexed
(D) Passive flexion until thigh meet with abdomen, associated with some degree of flexion of vertebral column

14. True statement regarding extension at hip joint is/ are:

(A) Range of extension beyond vertical line is about 40°- 50°
(B) Hyper extension is prevented by ilio- femoral ligament
(C) Head of femur occupy most superficial position in socket
(D) Extension makes joint loose packed condition

15. False statement regarding movement at hip joint is/ are:

(A) Adduction is limited by tension of the lateral band of ilio- femoral ligament
(B) Hyper extension is prevented by ilio- femoral ligament
(C) Flexion is limited to about 90°- 100° with extended knee joint
(D) In coxa vara abduction is more free in comparison to normal

16. During medial rotation on hip joint which movement occure when foot is on the ground:

(A) Medial femoral condyle rotate backward and simultaneously greater trochanter rotate forward

(B) Medial femoral condyle rotate forward and simultaneously greater trochanter rotate forward

(C) Medial femoral condyle rotate backward and simultaneously greater trochanter rotate backwad

(D) Medial femoral condyle rotate forward and simultaneously greater trochanter rotates backward

17. All muscles produce or help in flexion of hip joints except:

(A) Ilio – psoas

(B) Obturator internus

(C) Rectus femoris

(D) Sartorius

18. Extension at hip joint is produced by which muscle:

(A) Gluteus maximus

(B) Gluteus medius

(C) Gluteus minimus

(D) Rectus femoris

19. True statement regarding extension at hip joint is/ are:

(A) Gluteus maximus contracts when movement take place against resistance

(B) Hamstrings maintain extension in normal standing and walking

(C) Both are true statement

(D) None of above

20. All muscles produce adduction at hip joint except:

(A) Adductor longus

(B) Medial part of pectineus

(C) Gracilis

(D) Ischial part of adductor magnus

21. Abduction at hip joint is produced by:

(A) Anterior part of gluteus medius

(B) Gluteus maximus

(C) Long head of biceps femoris

(D) Vastus medialis

22. Medial rotator of hip joint is:

(A) Anterior fibers of gluteus medius

(B) Psoas major muscle when foot is off the ground

(C) Obturator externus

(D) Quadratus femoris

23. All are true regarding psoas major muscle except:

(A) It takes origin from iliac crest

(B) Gets inserted on lesser trochanter

(C) Acts as medial rotator when foot is on the ground

(D) Acts as lateral rotator when foot is off the ground

24. All are lateral rotator of hip joint except:

(A) Gluteus maximus

(B) Tensor fascia lata

(C) Obturator externus

(D) Quadratus femoris

25. Hip joint is supplied by all of following nerves except:

(A) Femoral nerve

(B) Anterior division of obturator nerve

(C) Inferior gluteal nerve

(D) Accessory obturator nerve

26. Coxa vara is a condition charecterized by:
(A) When neck shaft angle is increased
(B) Produce interference of action of gluteus maximus
(C) Cause marked limitation of abduction due to early impingement of greater trochanter on the ilium
(D) All of above

27. False statement regarding congenital dislocation of hip joint is/ are:
(A) More common in girls
(B) Due to vertical lateral wall of pelvis
(C) Femoral head is dislocated towards gluteal surface of ilium
(D) Abduction movement is limited

28. True statement regarding Nelton's line is/ are:
(A) Drawn by joining ASIS and ischial tuberosity
(B) Passes through the highest part of greater trochanter
(C) If greater trochanter is found to lie above or below line, some deformity of femoral neck is suspected
(D) All of above are true

29. All the arteries or its branches supply the hip joint except:
(A) Medial circumflex femoral artery
(B) Lateral circumflex femoral artery
(C) Superficial circumflex iliac artery
(D) Superior gluteal artery

30. All of muscle situated behind hip joint except:
(A) Obturator internus
(B) Quadratus femoris
(C) Gracilis
(D) Piriformis

31. Muscle situated anterior to hip joint is:
(A) Reflected head of rectus femoris
(B) Tensor fascia lata
(C) Psoas major
(D) Gemelli

32. Muscle present above the hip joint:
(A) Straight head of rectus femoris
(B) Gluteus minimus in the lateral part
(C) Obturator externus
(D) Piriformis

33. Structure is/ are situated in- front of hip joint:
(A) Trunk of femoral nerve in between ilicus and psoas
(B) Superior gluteal nerve and vessels
(C) Nerve to quadratus femoris
(D) Reflected head of rectus femoris

34. Structure is/ are present behind hip joint:
(A) Femoral artery in front of psoas tendon
(B) Straight head of rectus femoris
(C) Lateral part of pectineus
(D) Inferior gluteal nerve and vessels

35. All are structures situated anterior to hip joint except:
(A) Lateral part of pectineus
(B) Superior gluteal vessels
(C) Femoral artery in front of psoas tendon
(D) Straight head of rectus femoris

36. All are structure present posterior to hip joint except:
(A) Inferior gluteal vessels
(B) Sciatic nerve
(C) Femoral vessel
(D) Nerve to quadratus femoris

37. Knee joint is a type of joint:
(A) Ball and socket
(B) Condylar and modified hinge
(C) Saddle joint
(D) Ellipsoid and hinge variety

38. True statement regarding condyles of femur is/ are:
(A) Both condyle bulge backward
(B) Anterior surface of both condyles form patellar articular surface
(C) Patellar surface extends much higher over lateral femoral condyle
(D) All of above are true

39. Articular surfaces of femoral condyles are characterize by:
(A) Patellar surface of femur extends to under surface of medial femoral condyle
(B) Most medial facet of patella come in contact with semilunar impression of femur during full flexion of knee
(C) Lateral condyle of femur is more massive than medial
(D) All of above

40. Which of the following feature is/ are of lateral condyle of femur:
(A) Lateral epicondyle provide attachment to fibular collateral ligament
(B) A intracapsular curved groove present below epicondyle
(C) Lower and anterior part of groove gives origin to popliteus
(D) All of above

41. True statement regarding intercondylar notch of femur is/ are:
(A) Lateral wall of notch receive attachment of anterior cruciate ligament
(B) Medial wall of it gives attachment of posterior cruciate ligament
(C) Both 'a' and 'b' are true
(D) None of above

42. Tibial condyles are characterized by:
(A) Both are concave
(B) Much shallower than corresponding condyles of femur
(C) Both 'a' and 'b' are true
(D) None of above

43. Articular surfaces of tibial condyles is characterized by:
(A) Articular surface of medial condyle is ovoid
(B) Medial condylar surface is smaller antero- posteriorly then lateral
(C) Anterior margin of articular surface of lateral condyle grooved for tendon of popliteus
(D) All of above

44. The anterior part of intercondylar area gives attachment to the following before backward:
(A) Anterior horn of medial laminiscus, Lower attachment of anterior cruciate ligament, Anterior horn of lateral laminiscus
(B) Lower attachment of anterior cruciate ligament, Anterior horn of lateral laminiscus, Anterior horn of medial laminiscus
(C) Anterior horn of lateral laminiscus, Lower attachment of anterior cruciate ligament, Anterior horn of medial laminiscus
(D) Lower attachment of anterior cruciate ligament, Anterior horn of medial laminiscus, Anterior horn of lateral laminiscus

45. The posterior part of intercondylar area provide attachment to the following before backward:

(A) Posterior horn of lateral laminiscus, Posterior horn of medial laminiscus, Lower attachment of posterior cruciate ligament

(B) Posterior horn of medial laminiscus, Lower attachment of posterior cruciate ligament, Posterior horn of lateral laminiscus

(C) Lower attachment of posterior cruciate ligament, Posterior horn of medial laminiscus, Posterior horn of lateral laminiscus

(D) Posterior horn of medial laminiscus, Posterior horn of lateral laminiscus, Lower attachment of posterior cruciate ligament

46. Lateral condyle of tibia is characterized by:

(A) Postero lateral surface of it articulate with head of femur

(B) Anterior surface of it gives attachment to ilio tibial tract

(C) Both are true

(D) None of above

47. What happen of patella in full extension of knee joint:

(A) Lower two facet of patella come in contact with femur

(B) Middle two facet of it come in contact with femur

(C) The patella remain free from femur

(D) Medial most facet occupy semilunar area on medial femoral condyle

48. All are true regarding patella except:

(A) Largest sesamoid bone of body

(B) Ossified in tendon of quadriceps femoris

(C) When fractured easily get united

(D) Devoid of periosteum

49. Natural tendency of lateral displacement of patella is / are prevented by:

(A) Raised lateral margin of the patellar articular surface of femur

(B) Insertion of vastus medialis extends more below than insertion of vastus laterallis

(C) Both are true

(D) None of above

50. Functions of patella describes as:

(A) It is essential for movement of knee joint

(B) Facilitates the end of extension

(C) Help in beginning of extension from extreme flexion

(D) All of above

51. All are true statement regarding capsular ligament of knee joint:

(A) Deficient above patella

(B) Behind lateral condyle of tibia pierced by tendon of popliteus

(C) It strengthen posteriorly by oblique popliteal ligament

(D) All are true statements

52. Strengthening elements regarding capsular ligament of knee joint:

(A) Posteriorly by oblique popliteal ligament

(B) Medially tibial collateral ligament

(C) Anterlaterally lateral patellar retinaculum and ilio tibial tract

(D) All are true

53. Capsular ligament of knee joint is characterized by:

(A) Fibular collateral ligament separated from it by tendon of popliteus

(B) Anteromedially strengthen by lateral patellar retinaculum and ilio tibial tract

(C) Outer suface of it provide attachment to peripheral margins of medial menisci

(D) All of above

54. True statement regarding upper attachment of capsular ligament of knee joint is/ are:

(A) Posteriorly attach to upper margin of intercodylar notch

(B) Anteriorly above patellar articular surface of femur it is deficient

(C) Laterally include origin of popliteus

(D) All of above are true

55. Supra patellar bursa is characterized by:

(A) It is an non synovial pouch

(B) Communicate with knee joint cavity

(C) Situated infront of posterior surface of shaft of femur

(D) All of above

56. All are true regarding supra patellar bursa except:

(A) Apex of it kept in position by attachment of articularis genu muscle

(B) Situated between quadriceps femoris and anterior surface of lower part of shaft of femur

(C) Communicate with knee joint cavity

(D) None of above is true

57. Infra patellar fold is / are characterized by:

(A) A triangular fold of synovial membrane

(B) Extend upward and backward

(C) Intervene between the femoro-patellar and both condylar part of knee joint

(D) All are true

58. True statement regarding infra-patellar fold is/ are:

(A) Apex is attached to lower margin of intercondylar notch of femur

(B) Base is directed towards ligamentum patellae

(C) Lateral margins of it free and form alar fold

(D) All are true

59. Ligamentum patellae is characterized by:

(A) Derived from tendon of biceps femoris

(B) Extends from base of patella to condyle of tibia

(C) When knee is locked at end of extension all ligaments are taut except it

(D) All are true

60. Tibial collateral ligament is characterized by:

(A) It represent detached lower part of tendon of ischial fibres of adductor magnus

(B) Above it is attached to adductor tubercle on femoral condyle

(C) Superficial part of it blend with fibrous capsule

(D) All are true

61. True statement regarding tibial collateral ligament is /are :

(A) Above it is attached to medial epicondyle of femur

(B) Deep part of it blend with fibrous capsule

(C) Inferior medial genicular nerve and vessels lie between its deep and superficial part

(D) All are true

62. Fibular collateral ligament is characterized by:

(A) It extend as fibrous cord upward and forward

(B) Deep part of it blend with fibrous capsule

(C) Morphologically derived from primitive origin of peroneus longus muscle

(D) All are true

63. True statement regarding fibular collateral ligament is/ are:

(A) Extend from lateral epicondyle of femur to head of fibula

(B) It is overlapped superficially by tendon of biceps femoris

(C) Gap between ligament and capsule filled by tendon of popliteus

(D) All are true

64. Oblique popliteal ligament is characterized by:

(A) It is an expansion of insertion of semimembranosus

(B) Extend downward and medially from posterior surface of medial condyle of tibia

(C) Forms roof of popliteal fossa

(D) All are true

65. True statement regarding oblique popliteal ligament is/ are:

(A) Extend upward and laterally to lateral part of intercondylar line of femur

(B) Blend with posterior surface of the fibrous capsule

(C) Pierced by middle genicular nerve and vessels

(D) All are true

66. Arcuate ligament is characterized by:

(A) Anterior band arches over tendon of popliteus

(B) Forms Y shaped fibrous band

(C) Posterior band often deficient

(D) All are true

67. True statement regarding arcuate ligament of knee joint is/ are:

(A) Stem is fixed to styloid process of head of fibula

(B) Anterior band is attached to lateral condyle of femur

(C) Posterior band is attached to lateral condyle of tibia

(D) All are true

68. Cruciate ligaments are characterized by:

(A) They are intra synovial and extra capsular

(B) Named accordingly their femoral attachment

(C) Taut at extreme of flexion and extension

(D) All are true

69. True statement regarding cruciate ligament is/ are:

(A) They cross like the letter 'X'

(B) Developed from posterior part of primitive intercondylar septum

(C) Both are true

(D) None of above

70. True statement regarding anterior cruciate ligament is/ are:

(A) Below attached to anterior part of intercondylar area on tibia between anterior horn of medial and lateral menisci

(B) Above attached to posterior part of medial surface of lateral condyle of femur

(C) Oblique in direction and extend upward, backward and laterally

(D) All are true

71. All are function of anterior cruciate ligament except:

(A) Binds the bones together

(B) Stretched during flexion

(C) Prevent forward displacement of tibia

(D) In standing it lodge in notch in lateral part of intercondylar notch of femur

72. Posterior cruciate ligament is characterized by:

(A) Below attached to posterior part of intercondylar area of tibia behind posterior horns of medial and lateral menisci

(B) Above attached to anterior part of lateral surface of medial condyle of femur

(C) Extends upward, forward and medially

(D) All of above

73. All are functions of posterior cruciate ligament except:

(A) Both cruciate ligaments prevent side to side displacement of femur and tibia

(B) Binds the bones together

(C) Stretched during flexion

(D) Prevent forward displacement of tibia

74. True statement regarding menisco-femoral ligament is/ are:

(A) It connect posterior horn of lateral meniscus to medial condyle of femur

(B) Posterior ligament passes behind posterior cruciate ligament

(C) Regulates forward movement of lateral meniscus during extension

(D) All are true

75. True statement regarding menisci of knee joint:

(A) Composed of fibro cartilage

(B) Project from fibrous capsule as complete partition

(C) Intervene between condyles of femur and patella

(D) All are true

76. Characteristic features of medial menisci is / are:

(A) Semilunar in shape

(B) Antero- posteriorly longer than lateral one

(C) Attach to tibial collateral ligament

(D) All are true

77. Lateral menisci is characterized by:

(A) Forms 1/5 of a circle

(B) Anterior horn gives attachment to menisco- femoral ligament

(C) Popliteus prevent trapping of it at beginning of flexion

(D) All are true

78. True statement regarding menisci is/ are:

(A) Peripheral attached part of it avascular

(B) Inner free part gets nutrition from capsular arteries

(C) Act as shock absorber

(D) All are true

79. True statement about range of movement on knee joint is /are:

(A) The range of extension beyond vertical axis about 5°- 10°

(B) Range of flexion with extended hip about 120°

(C) Both are true

(D) None of above

80. All are flexors of knee joint except:

(A) Tensor fascia lata

(B) Semimembranosus

(C) Biceps femoris

(D) Sartorius

81. All are medial rotator of knee joint except:

(A) Semitendinosus

(B) Biceps femoris

(C) Gracilis

(D) Popliteus

82. Structure situated infront of knee joint:

(A) Medial patellar retinaculum

(B) Sartorius

(C) Quadriceps femoris

(D) Ilio- tibial tract

83. Structure form postero- lateral relation of knee joint:

(A) Tendon of biceps femoris

(B) Common peroneal nerve

(C) Both are true

(D) None of above

84. Structure situated antero- laterally to knee joint:

(A) Planteris

(B) Ilio- tibial tract

(C) Common peroneal nerve

(D) Sartorius

85. All are structures situated postero-medial to knee joint except:

(A) Gracilis

(B) Semitendinosus

(C) Tendon of biceps femoris

(D) Sartorius

86. All are structure situated behind knee joint except:

(A) Popliteal vessels

(B) Common peroneal nerve

(C) Both head of gastrocnemius

(D) Tibial nerve

87. Subcutaneous pre patellar bursa is characterized by:

(A) Intervene between skin and anterior surface of patella

(B) Also called house- maid's bursa

(C) Gets swollen by adopting kneel-down position during floor washing

(D) All are true

88. Subcutaneous infra- patellar bursa is characterized by:

(A) Intervene between skin and tubercle of tibia

(B) Swollen during praying in kneel down position with trunk upright

(C) Also called clergyman's bursa

(D) All are true

89. True statement regarding deep infra-patellar bursa:

(A) Intervene between patellar ligament and anterior surface of upper end of tibia

(B) Communicate with knee joint cavity

(C) Both are true

(D) None of above

90. All bursa are situated laterally to knee joint except:
(A) Between lateral head of gastrocnemius and the capsule
(B) Clergyman's bursa
(C) Between tendon of biceps femoris and fibular collateral ligament
(D) Between fibular collateral ligament and tendon of popliteus

91. All bursa communicate with knee joint cavity except:
(A) Supra- patellar bursa
(B) Bursa between medial head of gastrocnemius and the capsule
(C) Bursa between insertion of semimembranosus and medial condyle of tibia
(D) Bursa between fibular collateral ligament and tendon of popliteus

92. Knee joint is supplied by:
(A) Genicular branch of popliteal
(B) Descending genicular branch of femoral
(C) Descending branch of lateral circumflex femoral
(D) All are supplied joint

93. Which of following nerve is not a branch of tibial nerve:
(A) Superior medial genicular
(B) Inferior medial genicular
(C) Recurrent genicular
(D) Middle genicular

94. Knee joint is supplied by:
(A) Through nerve to the vastii
(B) Recurrent genicular
(C) Posterior division of obturator
(D) All of above

95. All are branches of common peroneal nerve except:
(A) Superior lateral genicular
(B) Inferior lateral genicular
(C) Middle genicular
(D) Recurrent genicular

96. Common structure get injured in knee joint:
(A) Medial menisci
(B) Fibular collateral ligament
(C) Posterior cruciate ligament
(D) Lateral menisci

97. ACL tear characterized by:
(A) Due to blow to anterior aspect of flexed knee
(B) Exhibit anterior displacement of tibia from femur in flexed knee
(C) Both are true
(D) None of above

98. More chances of injury in medial menisci than lateral is:
(A) Antero-posterior length is more in medial menisci than lateral
(B) Due to attachment of medial menisci to tibial collateral ligament
(C) Both are true
(D) None of above

99. Reason of lateral menisci is less commonly injured:
(A) Popliteus pull its posterior horn backward and prevent trapping between articular surfaces
(B) Menisco- femoral ligaments regulate forward gliding of it on tibial plateau during extension
(C) Both are true
(D) None of above

100. True statement regarding injury to cruciate ligaments:

(A) Most common variety of injury around knee joint

(B) Anterior cruciate ligament is more commonly injured than posterior

(C) Both are true

(D) None of above

101. All are true regarding patellar fracture except:

(A) Mostly caused by indirect violence

(B) Line of fracture passes transversely in most of cases

(C) Healing of fracture is very fast

(D) None of above

102. Superior tibio- fibular joint is characterized by:

(A) Syndesmosis variety of joint

(B) Supplied by Nerve to popliteus

(C) Help in planer flexion of the foot

(D) All are true

103. True statement regarding interosseous membrane between tibia and fibula is:

(A) Directed medially and downward in upper part

(B) Pierced by perforating branch of peroneal artery

(C) Both are true

(D) None of above

104. True statement regarding middle tibio- fibular joint is:

(A) Fibrous variety of joint

(B) Formed by crural interosseous membrane

(C) Membrane is continuous with interosseous ligament of inferior tibio fibular joint

(D) All are true

105. All of following structure situated infront of middle tibio fibular joint except:

(A) Tibialis anterior

(B) Anterior tibial vessels

(C) Flexor hallucis longus

(D) Deep peroneal nerve

106. All nerve supply inferior tibio fibular joint except:

(A) Deep peroneal nerve

(B) Superficial peroneal nerve

(C) Nerve to popliteus

(D) Tibial nerve

107. True statement regarding inferior tibio femoral joint is:

(A) Syndesmosis type of joint

(B) Supplied by common peroneal nerve

(C) All of ligaments of joint get relaxed during dorsi flexion

(D) All are true

108. True statement regarding posterior tibio fibular ligament is:

(A) Extends downward and laterally

(B) Few fibres of it continue with inferior transvers ligament

(C) Both are true

(D) None of above

109. Inferior transverse ligament is characterized by:

(A) Extends below articular surface

(B) Increase concavity of tibio fibular mortice of ankle joint

(C) Extends from malleolar fossa of fibula to posterior margin of lower end of tibia

(D) All are true

110. All are ligaments of inferior tibio fibular joint except:
(A) Anterior tibio fibular ligament
(B) Interosseous membrane
(C) Posterior tibio fibular ligament
(D) Interosseous ligament

111. Articular surfaces of talus is characterized by:
(A) Comma shape facet on medial side
(B) Triangular facet on lateral side
(C) Upper surface is broader in anterior part
(D) All are true

112. All structures form tibio fibular mortise in ankle joint except:
(A) Medial malleolus
(B) Posterior tibio fibular ligament
(C) Lateral malleolus
(D) Inferior transvers tibio femoral ligament

113. True statement regarding articular surfaces of ankle joint is/ are:
(A) Tip of Medial malleolus lies 2 cm below lateral
(B) Epiphyseal plate of lateral malle-olus correspond with joint space
(C) Upper surface of talus concave from before backward
(D) All are true

114. Capsular ligament of ankle joint is characterized by:
(A) It is thin in front and behind the joint
(B) Attached above to bone of tibio fibular mortise close to periphery of articular surface
(C) Below in anterior part extends to dorsal rough surface of neck of talus
(D) All are true

115. True statement regarding deltoid ligament is/ are:
(A) Triangular in shape
(B) Blends with fibrous capsule of ankle joint
(C) Consists of superficial and deep part
(D) All are true

116. Superficial part of deltoid ligament is characterized by:
(A) Apex is attached to tip of tibial malleolus
(B) Anterior part of it attach on navicular tuberosity
(C) Posterior part attach to medial tubercle of talus
(D) All are true

117. Deltoid ligament is characterized by:
(A) Deep part of it connect depression close to tip of tibial malleolus to medial surface of talus
(B) Ligament is crossed superficially by tendon of tibialis posterior
(C) Both are true
(D) None of above

118. Regarding anterior talo fibular ligament true statement is/ are:
(A) It is a strong band
(B) Extends from anterior margin of fibular malleolus to lateral surface of neck of talus
(C) Extends forward and laterally
(D) All are true

119. Posterior talo fibular ligament is characterized by:
(A) Extends backward and medially
(B) Extends from posterior margin of fibular malleolus to posterior tubercle of talus
(C) Both are true
(D) None of above

120. Calcaneo – fibular ligament is characterized by:
(A) Extends downward and backward
(B) Crossed superficially by tendon of peroneus longus and brevis
(C) Extends from notch near tip of fibular malleolus to elevation on lateral surface of calcaneus
(D) All of above are true

121. Natural tendency of forward dislocation of ankle joint is prevented by:
(A) Broader anterior part of trochlear surface of talus
(B) Tonic contraction of triceps surae through tendo- calcaneus
(C) Both are true
(D) None of above

122. Range of movement on ankle joint is:
(A) Dosiflexion is about 10°
(B) Planterflexion is about 20°
(C) Dorsiflexion when assisted by tarsal joints about 20°
(D) All range can possible

123. Which event occurred during dorsi flexion of ankle joint:
(A) Joint is in closed packed position
(B) Stretching of inferior tibio fibular joint
(C) Concomitant upward gliding movement of fibula at superior tibio fibular joint
(D) All movement occurred

124. Reason of dislocation of ankle joint during planter flexion:
(A) Joint is in closed packed condition
(B) Some space remain between tibio femoral mortise and narrow posterior part of trochlear surface of talus during movement
(C) Both are true
(D) None of above

125. Reason of slight planter flexion position during surgical immobilization:
(A) Because joint remain in close packed position
(B) Flushing of synovial fluid for nourishment of articular cartilage
(C) Both are true
(D) None of above

126. All muscle produce dorsiflexion at ankle joint except:
(A) Tibialis posterior
(B) Extensor digitorum longus
(C) Extensor hallucis longus
(D) Peroneus tertius

127. All muscle produce planter flexion at ankle joint except:
(A) Gastrocnemius
(B) Tibialis anterior
(C) Flexor digitorum longus
(D) Soleus

128. True statement regarding planter flexion at ankle joint is/ are:
(A) Soleus initiate the movement
(B) Gastrocnemius maintain the movement
(C) Peroneus longus and brevis come into play in extreme planter flexion
(D) All are true

129. All structure situated in front of ankle joint except:
(A) Tibialis anterior
(B) Flexor hallucis longus
(C) Anterior tibial vessels
(D) Deep peroneal nerve

130. All structures are present behind tibial malleolus except:
(A) Tibialis posterior
(B) Extensor digitorum longus
(C) Posterior tibial vessels
(D) Tibial nerve

131. True statement regarding tendons behind fibular malleolus:
(A) Tendon of peroneus longus and brevis
(B) Tendon of peroneus longus situated deep to brevis
(C) Both are true
(D) None of above

132. All arteries supply ankle joint except:
(A) Malleolar branch of anterior tibial
(B) Malleolar branch of posterior tibial
(C) Malleolar branch of peroneal
(D) All branch supply the joint

133. Pott's fracture is / are:
(A) Horizontal fracture of medial malleolus
(B) Oblique fracture of fibular shaft
(C) Both are component
(D) None of above

134. True statement regarding interphalangeal joints of foot:
(A) Example of typical hinge variety
(B) Possess capsular and collateral ligament
(C) Permit dorsi and planter flexion
(D) All are true

135. True statement regarding mid tarsal joint:
(A) Consists of 2 components with separated joint cavity
(B) Medially talo-calcano-navicular and laterally calcaneo-coboid
(C) Both are connected with bifurcated ligament
(D) All are true

136. In talo-calcaneo-navicular joint socket is formed by:
(A) Concave posterior surface of navicular bone
(B) Upper surface of planter calcaneonavicular ligament
(C) Anterior two talar facet on upper surface of sustenticulum tali
(D) All are collectively form

137. Planter calcaneo- navicular (spring) ligament is characterized by:
(A) Connect planter surface of navicular with sustenticulum tali
(B) Composed of elastic tissue
(C) Help in maintaining lateral longitudinal arch
(D) All are true

138. True statement regarding spring ligament is / are:
(A) Medially continuous with superficial fibres of deltoid ligament
(B) Laterally continuous with short planter ligament
(C) Both are true
(D) None of above

139. Lower surface of spring ligament is related to the muscle:
(A) Slip of tibialis posterior tendon
(B) Tendon of flexor digitorum longus
(C) Tendon of flexor hallusis longus
(D) All muscles are related

140. True statement regarding calcaneo cuboid joint:
(A) Saddle variety of joint
(B) Between anterior surface of calcaneous & posterior surface of cuboid
(C) Articular surfaces are concavo – convex and reciprocally curved
(D) All are true

141. True statement regarding bifurcated ligament is:
(A) Rectangular in shape
(B) Extend between talocalcaneo- navicular and calcaneo- cuboid joints
(C) Both are true
(D) None of above

142. Bifurcated ligament is characterized by:
(A) Y shape ligament
(B) Has calcaneo-navicular component
(C) Has calcaneo- cuboid component
(D) All are true

143. Attachments of bifurcated ligament is/ are:
(A) Stem attached to upper surface of anterior part of calcaneus
(B) Medially attach on dorsolateral aspect of navicular bone
(C) Laterally on dorsomedial aspect of cuboid
(D) All are attachments of ligament

144. True regarding short planter ligament is /are:
(A) Connect planter aspect of calcaneus in front of anterior tubercle to cuboid bone behind oblique ridge
(B) Situated below long planter ligament
(C) Both are true
(D) None of above

145. Long planter ligament is characterized by:
(A) Attached triangular area between anterior and two posterior tubercle to oblique ridge of cuboid
(B) Forms osseo- fibrous tunnel for tendon of peroneus longus
(C) Both are true
(D) None of above

146. Longest and strongest tarsal ligament is:
(A) Deltoid ligament
(B) Long planter ligament
(C) Spring ligament
(D) Bifurcated ligament

147. True statement regarding long planter ligament is / are:
(A) Situated below short planter ligament
(B) Maintain lateral longitudinal arch
(C) Attached to base of 2nd , 3rd and 4th metatarsal bone
(D) All are true

148. True statement regarding subtalar joint:
(A) Also called posterior talo-calcanean joint
(B) Modified multi- axial synovial joint
(C) Formed between articular facet on lower surface of body of talus and upper surface of middle third of calcaneus
(D) All are true

149. Interosseous talo-calcaneun ligament is characterized by:
(A) Fill up bony canal of sinus tarsi
(B) Seprate posterior talo- calcanean joint to talo- calcaneo- navicular joint
(C) Medial fibre of it are taut in eversion
(D) All are true

150. True statement regarding cervical ligament is/ are:
(A) Situated medial to interosseous ligament
(B) Connect upper surface of calcaneus to lateral surface of neck of talus
(C) Become taut during evesion
(D) All are true

Answersheet

1. **B**	2. **C**	3. **C**	4. **A**	5. **D**	6. **D**	7. **C**	8. **B**	9. **B**	10. **D**
11. **C**	12. **D**	13. **B**	14. **B**	15. **D**	16. **A**	17. **B**	18. **A**	19. **C**	20. **D**
21. **A**	22. **A**	23. **A**	24. **B**	25. **C**	26. **C**	27. **D**	28. **D**	29. **C**	30. **C**
31. **C**	32. **B**	33. **A**	34. **D**	35. **B**	36. **C**	37. **B**	38. **D**	39. **D**	40. **D**
41. **C**	42. **C**	43. **A**	44. **A**	45. **A**	46. **C**	47. **C**	48. **C**	49. **C**	50. **B**
51. **D**	52. **D**	53. **A**	54. **A**	55. **B**	56. **D**	57. **D**	58. **D**	59. **C**	60. **A**
61. **D**	62. **C**	63. **D**	64. **A**	65. **D**	66. **B**	67. **D**	68. **C**	69. **C**	70. **D**
71. **B**	72. **D**	73. **D**	74. **D**	75. **A**	76. **D**	77. **C**	78. **C**	79. **C**	80. **A**
81. **B**	82. **C**	83. **C**	84. **B**	85. **C**	86. **B**	87. **D**	88. **D**	89. **A**	90. **B**
91. **D**	92. **D**	93. **C**	94. **D**	95. **C**	96. **A**	97. **C**	98. **A**	99. **C**	100. **C**
101. **C**	102. **B**	103. **C**	104. **D**	105. **C**	106. **B**	107. **A**	108. **C**	109. **D**	110. **B**
111. **D**	112. **B**	113. **B**	114. **D**	115. **D**	116. **D**	117. **C**	118. **B**	119. **C**	120. **D**
121. **C**	122. **D**	123. **D**	124. **B**	125. **B**	126. **A**	127. **B**	128. **C**	129. **B**	130. **B**
131. **A**	132. **B**	133. **C**	134. **D**	135. **D**	136. **D**	137. **A**	138. **C**	139. **D**	140. **D**
141. **C**	142. **D**	143. **D**	144. **A**	145. **C**	146. **B**	147. **D**	148. **D**	149. **D**	150. **B**